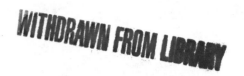

CAPTAIN OF DEATH

The Story of Tuberculosis

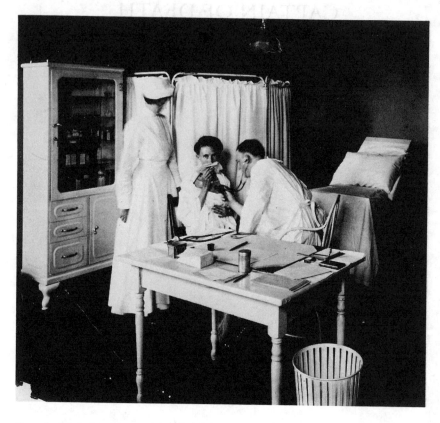

Frontispiece. A patient with tuberculosis being examined by his physician in about 1900. Little was available in the way of treatment for persons afflicted with tuberculosis at that time; the fortunate might find beds in sanatoria. Even with the best of care, about forty percent of them would die of their disease. Photograph courtesy of the American Lung Association.

CAPTAIN OF DEATH

The Story of Tuberculosis

Thomas M. Daniel

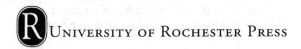
UNIVERSITY OF ROCHESTER PRESS

First published 1997
Reprinted in hardback and paperback 1999

University of Rochester Press
668 Mt. Hope Avenue
Rochester, NY 14620   USA

and at P.O. Box 9
Woodbridge, Suffolk IP12 3DF
United Kingdom

ISBN 1–878822–96–9 (Hardback)
ISBN 1–58046–070–4 (Paperback)

Library of Congress Cataloging-in-Publication Data

Daniel, Thomas M.
    Captain of death : the story of tuberculosis / Thomas M. Daniel.
        p.   cm.
    Includes index.
    ISBN 1–878822–96–9 (alk. paper)
    1. Tuberculosis—History. I. Title.
    [DNLM: 1. Tuberculosis—history.   WF 11.1 D184c 1997]
    RC311.D25   1997
    616.9′95′009—dc21
    DNLM/DLC
    for Library of Congress   97–29886
                                                                          CIP

British Library Cataloguing-in-Publication Data
A catalogue record for this book is
available from the British Library

Designed and typeset by Cornerstone Composition Services
Printed in the United States of America
This publication is printed on acid-free paper

For my wife Janet, whom I love dearly.
She has encouraged me and supported me not only
through the writing of this book but through a career
devoted to the study of tuberculosis.
And she is my best friend.

Pray, of what disease did Mr. Badman die? For I now perceive we are come up to his death.

I cannot so properly say that he died of one disease, for there were many that had consented, and laid their heads together, to bring him to his end. He was dropsical, he was consumptive, he was surfeited, was gouty, and, as some say, he had a tang of the foul distemper in his bowels. Yet the captain of all these men of death that came against him to take him away was the consumption, for it was that that brought him down to the grave.

The Life and Death of Mr. Badman
John Bunyan[1]

Contents

Introduction

One-third of the population of the world is infected with the germ that causes tuberculosis. Eight million people develop this disease each year. Ninety-five percent of them live and suffer in developing countries, only one-quarter of one percent of them in North America. Only one in five of the world's victims of tuberculosis receives adequate treatment. These awesome figures are increasing, year by year, and will almost certainly continue to increase.[2]

Tuberculosis killed St. Francis of Assisi. It killed Fédéric Chopin, Charlotte Brontë, George Orwell, and Eleanor Roosevelt. As we enter the third millennium of the common era, tuberculosis kills about two and one-half to three million people each year. It accounts for seven percent of the deaths in the world and more than one in four of the preventable deaths. Tuberculosis kills more people five years of age or older than AIDS, malaria, leprosy, and other tropical diseases combined. Among infections, this preventable and treatable disease is the number one killer in the world. It is truly the Captain of Death.

This book tells the story of tuberculosis. It does so by interweaving history, biography, and information about the nature of the disease. Consider the warp threads of the tuberculosis tapestry as time, stretching from the earliest historical records of human existence to the present and beyond. This book uses as its weft stories about people, people who had tuberculosis, people who fought to conquer tuberculosis. Those who weave tapestries use many colors of weft threads, and the many lives of persons who suffered from or studied tuberculosis provide many colors for my threads. So also do the many facets of the nature of this complex disease.

And the stories of people who had tuberculosis add more than colors to my weaving. They add challenges. Why did Eleanor Roosevelt live five decades with her tuberculosis germs trapped within her defender cells, the germs only to break out and ultimately kill her? How could this killer disease have stricken John Keats so fulminantly and yet produced smoldering, indolent illness in Robert Louis Stevenson? Josephine Baker and George Orwell both contracted tuberculosis during the decade just before effective drug treatment was discovered. Deprived of these miracle drugs by history, Baker recovered uneventfully but Orwell died. Why?

On a larger scale, what can we learn from tuberculosis in mummies both in Egypt and Peru? The mutinous crew of HMS Bounty escaped British law by fleeing to Pitcairn Island. When tuberculosis reached them it exacted a more severe punishment upon them and their descendants than any admiralty courts would have. How? And why did the enormous tuberculosis epidemic recede in Europe and North America before the institution of control measures and effective treatments? We in the biomedical professions now have ideas and theories, sometimes even facts, bearing on some of these questions. We also have still greater challenges as yet unmet.

This book is organized into four parts, each part a separate tapestry telling the story from a different viewpoint. Thus, this book first tells the story of tuberculosis in terms of its epidemiologic history through time. Next, the book recounts the story of the infectious nature of tuberculosis by tracing the history of the unfolding of knowledge of this important aspect of the disease. Then, in similar fashion, this book reveals the evolution of our knowledge of the resistance of people to tuberculosis. Finally, this volume describes the development of modern treatment. In each of these parts, the interweaving of accounts of people's lives and of the emergence of knowledge about tuberculosis is allowed to build the fabric of the story. A chronology presented in Appendix I and an index help the reader relate events in one section to those in others.

My tapestry—this book—is intended for general readers. I have tried to avoid technical and medical terms. When they seemed essential, I have tried to define them. Additionally, I have provided a glossary in Appendix II, which defines them in terms relevant to their use in this book.

I first met tuberculosis as an accident of an army assignment towards the end of the Korean War. Having finished my training in internal medicine and deferred my military obligation while I did so, I entered the army. Shortly thereafter, I found myself responsible for the care of a ward full of patients with tuberculosis at Valley Forge Army Hospital. After leaving the army and pursuing advanced training in microbiology and immunochemistry, I directed a research laboratory studying the tubercle bacillus and the response of patients to this organism. I interrupted my thirty year teaching and laboratory research academic career with a stint with the Peace Corps in Bolivia supervising and planning tuberculosis control programs, and I followed this with other experiences in the international arena, including consultancies to International Child Care in Haiti stretching over nearly a quarter of a century. I conducted research studies in Bolivia, Argentina, Mexico, and Uganda. I became fascinated with tuberculosis, and I devoted four exciting decades of my life to studying it.

There are many persons who deserve my thanks for leading me on the path of my studies of tuberculosis and for guiding and supporting me when I seemed to be wandering onto interesting detours less traveled by. Stephen Berté and William Dunnington, my commanding officers at Valley Forge, and Robert H. Ebert, my department chairman and mentor as I began my academic life, merit special mention as important persons who stimulated me early in my career to pursue my interest and curiosity about tuberculosis.

Abram B. Stavitsky made me a laboratory scientist. Austin S. Weisberger and Oscar D. Ratnoff continued that transformation. As my research career developed, I had many associates working in the laboratory with me. It would be impossible for me to acknowledge all of them, but Lavenia Ferguson, Ma Yu, Alamelu Raja, Rodney Benjamin, and Patricia Anderson certainly deserve my recognition and thanks. In the greater community of scholars of tuberculosis, Bernard W. Janicki, Sotiros D. Chaparas, and Patrick Brennan encouraged me, criticized my work, and helped me in uncounted ways.

C. William Keck and Gino Baumann seduced me to Bolivia and an epiphany in my life. Luis Valverde, Laura Pinell, and Graciela Murillo kept me returning to the land that became my *segunda patria*. And in Haiti, Marie Bellande has been a shining inspiration.

I recall with gratitude many additional colleagues in the academic, medical, microbiological, and public health communities at Case Western Reserve University and in Cleveland, the United States, and the world—friends and critics—who throughout my career have continued to stimulate me, sometimes disputing my ideas, sometimes supporting my thinking. Important among them in Cleveland have been Joseph B. Stocklen, Frits van der Kuyp, Emanuel Wolinsky, Gerald L. Baum, Scott R. Inkley, Jerrold J. Ellner, and Frederick C. Robbins. On the wider scene, there are too many individuals to mention, but Dennis Mitchison, Stefan Grzybowski, George Comstock, Joseph Bates, William Stead, Dixie Snider, and Philip Hopewell need special mention. The danger in any list of ackowledgements such as this is that someone has been omitted. In fact, I have surely omitted many, and I apologize to them.

My wife and my children have encouraged my interest, tolerated my weekend trips to the lab to check on important experiments, put up with my wanderings and often accompanied me as I pursued tuberculosis to remote corners of the earth, and provided life's leavening.

This book has been germinating in my mind for many years. I have collected the anecdotes and references that it contains from many sources over many years. I have done my best to verify them, and the notes to the text provide appropriate references. I am, first and last, a student of tuberculosis—not really an historian. For the most part, this book is constructed from secondary rather than primary sources, as will be evident to those who read the notes carefully. None-the-less, I have tried to be scholarly and accurate in all that I have written. In so far as possible—and it has almost always been possible—I have read the original papers cited in this work. When occasionally my reading has led me to doubts, I have expressed these doubts in the notes. Similarly, I have tried to annotate conflicting accounts of some historical events. The library resources of Case Western Reserve University, the Allen Medical Library, and the Cuyahoga County Library System have been invaluable to me, and I thank the many librarians who have encouraged me and assisted me in my wanderings through sometimes ancient volumes in library stacks.

My wife, Janet S. Daniel, Edward A. Nardell, and Baron Lerner each read the entire manuscript and made helpful comments and suggestions for revision. Sean M. Culhane of the University of Rochester Press has been helpful and encouraging as I brought this manuscript to fruition. I gratefully acknowledge his assistance.

Thomas M. Daniel, MD
Cleveland, Ohio

PART I

Consumption:
Tuberculosis Through the Ages

The Lord will smite you with consumption, and with fever, inflammation, and fiery heat, and with drought, and with blasting, and with mildew; and they shall pursue you until you perish.

Deuteronomy 28:22[1]

1

An Egyptian Girl; A Peruvian Boy

She died coughing blood, a victim of tuberculosis—unsung, unheralded, uncelebrated—not the darling of her era, not remembered in song like Violetta, La Traviata, but none-the-less lost. We do not know her name. She lived three thousand years ago in a crowded and dirty village along the Nile river near the present day Egyptian town of Dra Abu El-Naga.

She was a sickly child, feverish and fussy as an infant, slow in her development, yet loved by her parents. At an early age she developed a hunched back, and by the time she was five years old, it was apparent to everyone that she would not live long. Her parents took her to priests, who performed incantations, but told her parents that the consumption was an evil for which the gods offered few cures; there was little hope for their child. The young girl died in a fit of coughing, with blood coming from her mouth and nose, a victim of tuberculosis. Her parents wrapped her body in cloth and buried her in the tomb of Nebwenenef, a priest who had died three hundred years earlier. Maybe he could help their young daughter in her after-life journey.[2]

Perhaps on the same day or in the same year, certainly about the same time, in nearby Thebes, tuberculosis claimed a more prominent victim, Nesperehân, a high priest of Ramses. He also had tuberculosis of the spine and with it the hunchback deformity seen in Figure 1.1. His life had been one of opulence, and he was buried in a rich tomb.[3]

For both the nameless girl and the priest Nesperehân, the archeologic evidence for tuberculosis is strong. Indeed, typical tubercle bacilli were identified microscopically in the spine of the girl. These two individuals were not unusual cases in their time. Tuberculosis of the spine is abundantly portrayed in Egyptian art beginning about 3000 BCE. Many skeletons and mummies show evidence of this disease. It is thought by

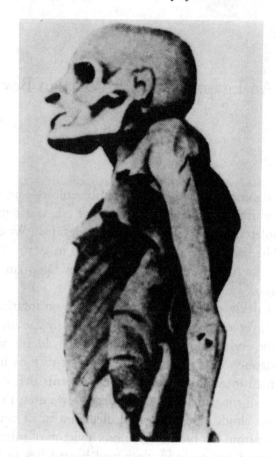

Figure 1.1. Mummy of the Egyptian priest Nesperehân, XXIst dynasty, about 1000 BCE. This mummy demonstrates the sharply angled, mid thoracic gibbous deformity characteristic of tuberculosis of the spine. The mummy also had a large psoas abscess, another characteristic form of chronic tuberculosis. Morse D, Brothwell DR, Ucko PJ. Tuberculosis in ancient Egypt. Amer Rev Respir Dis 1964; 90:524-41. Figure reproduced with permission of the American Lung Association.

some that deformed persons were valued as slaves in ancient Egypt, and perhaps persons with spinal tuberculosis were brought into Egypt from other parts of Africa. Perhaps also, early Egyptian artists chose to portray these odd-looking hunchback persons more frequently than they were truly present in the community.

Tuberculosis has many forms, but it is bony disease that is most easily recognized by archeologists, because it is bone that survives through history for modern scientists to study. And it is the typical hunchback of tuberculosis that is easily portrayed in art and recognized today. The hunched back of tuberculosis, sometimes called a gibbous deformity, is distinctive and different from the kyphoscoliosis deformity seen more commonly in North America and Europe today, which develops during adolescent growth, particularly in young women. As tuberculosis invades the spine, it destroys the anterior portions of the vertebral bodies, causing them to collapse forward. The result is a sharply angulated spinal deformity without twisting and with the shoulders remaining level. On the other hand, kyphoscoliotic disease causes twisting of the spine and drooping of one shoulder.

However easily it is recognized in art and skeletons, bony tuberculosis is not as common as the much more familiar lung disease. Today, bone disease represents only a few percent of cases of tuberculosis, and a high frequency of skeletal disease must mean an even higher frequency of lung disease. There can be little doubt that tuberculosis was common in predynastic and early dynastic Egypt.

In about 700 CE, more than a thousand years after the young Egyptian girl died but long before Columbus and Pizarro blazed the conquistador trail to Incan gold, a Nazca boy about ten years old died and was buried near Hacienda Agua Salada in Peru. He had tuberculosis of the lungs, liver, kidney, surface of the heart, and spine. As in the case of the Egyptian girl, tuberculosis germs were present in his tissues. This boy's mummified body was found seated on a cushioned adobe seat, a most unusual finding in Peruvian graves, and he appeared to have the shrunken legs of someone whose lower body is paralyzed. Such paralysis is a well recognized complication of tuberculosis of the spine. Someone cared for and provided a special seat for the crippled child.[4]

In 1994, scientists from Minnesota reported studies of a mummy from the arid desert region of southern Peru.[5] The mummy, dated to between 1000 and 1300 CE, was that of a woman in her early forties. Although she probably did not die of her tuberculosis, her lungs showed clear evidence of the disease. Using modern molecular biological techniques of polymerase chain reaction amplification, the North American scientists isolated DNA of the tubercle bacillus from her tuberculous lung lesions. Among one hundred and forty mummies studied from the Peruvian tomb site, one had tuberculosis. If one wishes to extrapolate from those numbers, then seven tenths of one percent of ancient Peruvians might have had this disease, making it common by modern standards in that remote corner of the world.

As in ancient Egypt, the hunchback deformity of tuberculosis of the spine is easily recognized in prehistoric art from the Americas. Carlos Ponce Sanginés described scores of prehistoric stone figures with probable tuberculosis of the spine from the preIncan site of Tiwanaku in Bolivia and elsewhere.[6] Several pieces clearly depicting spinal tuberculosis are on exhibit in the outstanding collection of the Museo Nacional de Antropología in Mexico City. Eight percent of figures on display at the Museo Popol-Vuh in Guatemala dating from approximately 300 BCE to 600 CE have deformed spines suggesting tuberculosis, and the geographic distribution of pieces with this deformity is not homogeneous, suggesting that some prehistoric communities had much more tuberculosis than others. There are no deformities represented from Petén while ten percent of figures from two other communities depict deformities that might represent spinal tuberculosis.[7]

Early writings of the Spanish conquistadores in Mexico describe the selection of hunchbacks as subjects for religious human sacrifice.[8] This parallels the apparent special status attributed to slaves with this disease in ancient Egypt. It might also be a factor in the high frequency of this form of tuberculosis in pre-Columbian American art.

Bernardo Arriaza and his colleagues had the opportunity to study nearly five hundred prehistoric mummies and skeletons from northern Chile representing a thirty-five hundred year period beginning in about 2000 BCE.[9] They found evidence of skeletal tuberculosis in five of their specimens, a high overall prevalence of one percent. However, as with the carved stone figures from Guatemala, the distribution was not uniform. In this case only one geographic site was involved, but there was variation over time. All of the tuberculous skeletons were dated to the first millennium CE, during which the prevalence was greater than two percent. Unlike representations in art, this extraordinarily high rate of occurrence cannot represent a preference of artisans for carving deformed persons.

So it is that from both Egypt and Peru we have incontrovertible evidence of the existence of tuberculosis in prehistoric times. How did it begin?

Human beings first appeared in the Rift Valley of Africa millions of years ago. We know very little about these early people. They hunted and gathered their food in small family groups of one or two dozen individuals. Their dialectic language groups, within which they probably found their mates, were larger, perhaps numbering a few hundred. As we will see shortly, populations of this size might have supported tuberculosis; we do not know if they did. Hundreds of thousands or perhaps a million years ago, these early humans began to move out of central Africa. They migrated, wandering in search of food and shelter, and their descendants peopled the earth. At some point, at some time, some of them developed tuberculosis. What we know of the disease in both the Nile valley and the Americas suggests that tuberculosis exploded in an epidemic involving large numbers of these early humans at about the time that agrarian societies developed. However, even before stable communities developed, hunters and gatherers were on the move, migrating to new lands, and taking tuberculosis with them as they peopled the world.

Inhabitants of India consecrated a hymn to the cure of "yakshma," which appears to have been tuberculosis, in about 2000 BCE. The causes of tuberculosis were thought to include over-fatigue, sorrow, fasting, and pregnancy. These ideas were prescient, for we now know that fatigue, depression, and pregnancy can all compromise cellular immunity to tuberculosis. The "Ordinances of Manu," written in India about 1300 BCE, warned against marriage into a family in which there was tuberculosis. The disease was one of lower castes, and a Brahmin prayer from that time intoned, "Oh Fever, with thy Brother Consumption, with thy Sister Cough, go to the people below."[10] Eight hundred years later, Sushruta Samhita described tuberculosis and considered it incurable. Physicians were advised not to treat this illness in order to protect their reputations.

Ancient Chinese literature used the term "laoping" to describe a lung disease that was probably tuberculosis. The art of moxa or moxibustion, in which burning tinder from dried leaves of mugwort was applied to specific points of the skin, was used in China to treat tuberculosis three thousand years ago. The ancient Chinese text Yüeh Ling

(Monthly Ordinances), which was probably written about the third century BCE, described "chiai nio." This chronic wasting disease caused patients to spit blood. It was almost certainly tuberculosis. One of the most famous physicians of early China was Shunyü. He was asked by a prince to examine the royal hand maidens. He identified one young woman who appeared to be well as suffering from "shang phi." Six months later she died while coughing blood.

The journey of early migrating people across what is now the Bering Strait but was then the Bering land bridge between Siberia and Alaska took place between eleven and twenty-five thousand years ago, chiefly in two or three waves.[11] The crippled Peruvian boy who died of tuberculosis hundreds of years before Europeans reached his country tells us that those early wanderers carried tuberculosis with them to the western hemisphere. En route, probably at some much earlier time and perhaps as long as twenty-five thousand years ago, the boy's more ancient ancestors had carried tuberculosis from Africa to Asia.

Some experts believe that most early human tuberculosis was contracted from tuberculosis in cattle.[12] Certainly, cattle develop this disease, usually caused by a special bovine type of tubercle bacilli, and cattle may transmit the bovine organism to people in whom it can also cause tuberculosis. Predynastic Egyptians domesticated cattle, and the young girl who died three thousand years ago might have lived in the same crude building with her family's cows and might have drunk contaminated milk. In fact, bovine tubercle bacilli appear to have a propensity for causing bone disease, and the large numbers of hunchbacks in prehistoric art might be more easily explained if bovine tubercle bacilli were common in those ancient times.

The amplification technique used to detect DNA of tuberculosis germs in a Peruvian mummy does not distinguish between human and bovine forms of the bacillus, but it is unlikely that bovine strains of tuberculosis were present in the Western Hemisphere in those early times. Cattle did not exist in North America until they were brought there by the Spaniards. Rarely, llamas acquire bovine tuberculosis, and these ancient camelids, which evolved in South America after its land mass split from the primitive continent of Gondwana some one hundred and sixty million years ago, were domesticated by early humans in South America. Dwellers in the high Andean regions also domesticate guinea pigs, often keeping them in their homes. These small animals readily contract tuberculosis, but they are more susceptible to human than bovine strains of the tubercle bacillus. However, no domesticated animals susceptible to bovine tuberculosis were present in North America, which the early wanderers crossed and also populated and where skeletal remains also demonstrate ancient tuberculosis. The Peruvian boy is unlikely to have caught his disease from an animal, and his hunched back was probably caused by a human type of tubercle bacillus.

Some historians have carried this argument to the point of suggesting that present day human tubercle bacilli evolved from bovine strains, which are similar to and in some ways simpler than human strains in their gene structure. It is more likely, however, that modern human and bovine tuberculosis germs have their origins in a shared primitive common ancestor, perhaps one that also infected some of the early humans' primate contemporaries. Most of the members of the genus of organisms to which this bacterium belongs live in soil and water, and only a few of them have evolved into germs that produce disease in people or animals. Those that do probably underwent their evolutionary change to become parasites of human beings at a distant time long before the earliest human archeologic records. Without denying the fact that bovine organisms may have caused disease in some early people, it now seems most likely that the bacteria that caused tuberculosis in most early people were members of the same species that infects people today.

In North America, the early people of the Mississippi and Ohio River valleys settled in small communities. Their burial grounds also yield evidence of tuberculosis, albeit not as dramatically as those in Egypt and Peru. The Jesuits, who first contacted the indigenous people of North America, clearly described individuals with tuberculosis. Based in part on studies of these North American populations and in part on mathematical simulations, we can estimate that a community size of between roughly two and four hundred persons is necessary for tuberculosis to become established in a population without either disappearing from the community or progressing to the point of killing all of the community members.[13] Viewed from the perspective of the parasite, success means infecting enough people to continue germ reproduction and proliferation without killing too many of the parasitized people who provide homes and sustenance for the germs. Early North Americans lived in groups of the size tuberculosis-causing microbes need to succeed, a similar size to the dialectic groups of their earlier African progenitors.

A modern parallel to the very early communities in which tuberculosis probably first became established exists today in the Mato Grosso region of Brazil. Isolated by impenetrable wet lands and protected by the Brazilian government, the tribes of the Mato Grosso still have little contact with one another and are rarely in contact with modern Brazil. I participated in a survey conducted by the Brazilian government and United States Peace Corps staff and volunteers in preparation for establishing health care programs for these people. We estimated the tuberculous infection rates in eleven villages, all with fewer than two hundred and fifty people. In some villages, more than eighty percent of the residents were infected. In others, no one was infected, and the tubercle bacillus was probably on the way to extinction. In one, only ten villagers survived, of whom nine were sick with tuberculosis; those villagers would soon be extinct.[14] This modern experience parallels the apparently scattered occurrence of tuberculosis among ancient Mayans as reflected in Guatemala's Museo Popol-Vuh.

The story of tuberculosis occurring in a patch work fashion has been repeated throughout history in various regions of the world, sometimes on scales as small as those of the Mato Grosso, sometimes on much larger scales. Early European explorers in Africa, the Pacific, and the Arctic did not frequently encounter tuberculosis in the people they contacted, and they found many communities in which this disease was unknown. In fact, it is likely that these early adventurers brought tuberculosis to many of the earth's uninfected indigenous peoples. Upon its arrival, tuberculosis often and tragically spread rapidly through these previously healthy peoples. At the same time, as we shall see later, tuberculosis was extraordinarily common in western Europe.

The Egyptian girl and the Peruvian boy died of a disease undiagnosed and mysterious to their parents and the priests or shamans who tried to help them. More advanced cultures and more advanced science would be needed before this disease, arguably the most important disease of human history, would be known and understood by medical practitioners. Centuries would pass in the discovery of that knowledge and acquisition of that understanding.

2

Kos, Alexandria, and Rome

A golden age of art and knowledge that spanned nearly a millennium surrounding the birth of Christ began in Greece and later spread to Alexandria and then to Rome. Interest in and knowledge of medicine flourished in Greece and later moved with Greek culture. Tuberculosis was known to those Greek physicians, and their writings give us further insights into the history of this disease.

In those peerless times of Greece and Rome, tuberculosis was well recognized, and we can read elegant descriptions of it written by the physicians of that era. They called it phthisis, φθίσις. The derivation of that word is not clear.[1] It may come from the ancient Greek word meaning to spit, φθυειν or φθυσις. Alternatively, phthisis may derive from φθίνειν, an ancient Greek word meaning to consume; consumption is the old testament biblical name for tuberculosis and the word still used in modern Bibles to translate *schanhepheth*, the ancient and modern Hebrew word for tuberculosis. Jehovah said to the Israelites ". . . I will even appoint over you terror, consumption, and the burning ague . . ." Later the wandering Israelites are exhorted to follow the law or "the Lord will smite you with consumption, and with fever, inflammation, and with heat . . . ; they shall pursue you until you perish"[2] It is quite clear from the context of their use that these ancient terms were used to describe tuberculosis, and both phthisis and consumption have persisted into recent, if not current or modern, English as names for tuberculosis.

Close to Turkey in the Aegean Sea, the Greek island of Kos was a famous health spa when Hippocrates was born there in about 460 BCE. Kos became the site of the temple to Asklepias, a legendary Greek physician who was elevated to be a god and considered the son of Apollo. A guild of physician families known as the Asklepiads was established on

Kos. Hippocrates' father, a physician, belonged to the guild, and Hippocrates followed the usual pattern of apprenticing himself to his father and joining the guild. He later traveled to Athens to further his studies of medicine.

We know surprisingly little about the man, Hippocrates. He wrote prolifically and he taught many others his art. He became famous in his day, and upon his death the Egyptian Pharaoh Ptolomy Soter charged his court scholars with writing a compendium of all of Hippocrates' writings. These savants included in their work a great deal of material from those associated with Hippocrates. Thus, it is hard to know with certainty what Hippocrates wrote and what others of the early Greek medical guild of Kos wrote.

Hippocrates and his fellow Asklepiads took medicine out of the realm of religion and the priesthood. Medicine became based on knowledge and science, not on religious tenets and superstitions. Disease was not due to acts of perverse gods. As exemplified by the Hippocratic oath, physicians became viewed as public servants and skilled craftsmen. Hippocrates was the first teacher of bedside medicine. He emphasized for the first time the need to examine the patient. In this sense, Hippocrates was indisputably the father of modern medicine.

Hippocrates knew tuberculosis well. He described it in its several forms, and some credit him with coining the name phthisis. He thought it was caused by growths in the lungs, which he termed tubercula, φυματα. Hippocrates noted the association of tuberculosis of the spine, the disease of the Egyptian priest Nesperehân, with pulmonary tuberculosis. In *Book I, Of the Epidemics*, Hippocrates wrote, "Consumption was the most considerable of the diseases which then prevailed, and the only one which proved fatal to many persons. Most of them were affected by these diseases in the following manner: fevers . . . , constant sweats, but not over the whole body, . . . sputa small, dense, concocted, but brought up rarely and with difficulty . . . they were soon wasted. So much concerning the phthisical afflictions."[3] These features—fever, sweats over the upper but not lower body, cough productive of little or no sputum, and wasting—are signs of tuberculosis still taught to medical students today.

Hippocrates was famous for his aphorisms. He wrote, "Consumption occurs chiefly between the ages of eighteen and thirty-five." This age distribution pattern of disease occurrence is typical of populations where tuberculosis is highly prevalent, and it often distinguishes highly prevalent populations from those where tuberculosis is receding and no longer common. From Hippocrates' statement alone, we can deduce that the ancient Greeks among whom Hippocrates lived, taught, and served as a doctor were a people with a great deal of consumption—tuberculosis.

Plato was born in 430 BCE and was a contemporary of Hippocrates. He advised against treating tuberculosis. He considered it untreatable, and wrote of treatment for consumption that "it was of no advantage to themselves nor to the State."

The Greeks ruled the world they knew, and Alexander the Great led his warriors across the eastern Mediterranean region. In 331 BCE, one year before his death, Alexander founded the city of Alexandria near the mouth of the Nile on the north coast of Egypt. Its famous library fostered learning and Alexandria became a center of scholarship. Herophilus (circa 300 BCE) and Erasistratus (circa 310-250 BCE) founded a medical school there about 50 years later. This school became the preeminent medical center of its era, and it was Greek physicians with their medical art who reigned there.

Areteus was a Greek physician who lived in Alexandria about the second century CE. He wrote of patients with tuberculosis that those "most prone to phthisis are the slender, those whose scapulae are like wings or folding doors, those who have prominent throats, who are pale, and have narrow chests."[4] This relationship of asthenic stature with tuberculosis is a theme persisting throughout history, and in fact, modern data demonstrate that those who are somewhat overweight are less likely to contract this disease. Areteus also wrote with great insight into the physical and mental state of his tuberculous patients, "Hemorrhage from the lungs is particularly dangerous, although patients do not despair even when near their end. The insensibility of the lungs to pain appears to me to be the cause of this, for pain is more dreadful than precarious; whereas in the absence of it, even serious illness is unaccompanied by fear of death and is more dangerous than dreadful."[5]

Although tuberculosis was well known to the Greek physicians at Alexandria, it is apparent that it was not their major concern. One can deduce from the fact that they wrote little about it that it was not the frequently encountered problem that it was in Greece itself—certainly not the scourge that it was in the Nile Valley in early dynastic times. The epidemic of tuberculosis in Egypt appears to have waned by the time of the height of Alexandrian civilization.

As Rome became ascendent in the classical world, it was Greek physicians who provided medical care for Caesar's armies. The renowned Greek physician Asklepiades arrived in Rome in 91 BCE; he was skilled and he quickly gained acceptance for Greek medicine. Previously, the Roman ruler Cato had tried to keep all doctors out of Rome. Then, in 46 BCE Julius Caesar granted Roman citizenship to all physicians.

Clarissimus Galenus was born in the Greek city of Pergmon in Asia Minor in 131 CE. His father, Nikon, was an accomplished mathematician and architect. When young Galen was seventeen, his father had a visionary dream and following the instructions received in this dream enrolled his son in the study of medicine. Galen was a brilliant student. He continued his studies in Smyrna, and by age twenty-one he was a well known doctor and he had written books on obstetrics, eye disease, and pulmonary disease. At age twenty-eight he was appointed physician to the gladiators in the local stadium.

In 162 CE, Galen went to Rome. While he found the busy city fascinating and stimulating, he had only scorn and sarcasm for Roman physicians and the various sects with their conflicting theories of medicine to which they belonged. Galen wrote of the contemporary Roman medical scene, "the greatest flatterer, not he who is the most skilled in the art, receives all advantages and finds all doors open." By 166 CE Galen had outlasted his welcome in Rome, and he fled before the criticism of the established medical sects.

Galen's exile from Rome was a temporary one, for he was well known to important people. The Emperor Marcus Aurelius called him back to help deal with a city besieged by a devastating plague. In 174 CE he was called upon to treat the Emperor himself for a stomach ailment. He put aside the foul tasting potions recommended by others and treated Marcus Aurelius with a warm wool pack on his stomach. The emperor recovered after this simple therapy, akin to a hot water bottle wrapped in a towel. Galen's writings persisted for centuries after his death, and it was a rare physician who sought to challenge his writings and teachings.

Galen recognized tuberculosis. He also recognized that it had many forms and he felt that it was infectious. The treatment he recommended was simple and homey—like the warm pack for the emperor's stomach. He prescribed fresh milk, open air, sea voyages, and dry elevated places. It would be a long time before medicine would find treatment for tuberculosis more efficacious than Galen's prescription.

What can we infer of tuberculosis in classical Rome? As one peruses the writings of the Greek physicians working there, it is apparent that they knew this disease. It is also evident that they were more interested in many other diseases and that tuberculosis was much less important to them than it had been to their predecessors in Greece. Probably tuberculosis was not common among the citizens of ancient Rome. Had it been prevalent previously and then declined as appears to have happened in Egypt? Or did it never become widespread? We cannot know the answer to that question. However, as will become apparent, tuberculosis epidemics do fade on their own. And, as we have seen, tuberculosis may be prevalent in one population and almost unknown in others of the same era.

3

The Middle Ages and Beyond

The roughly one thousand years that followed the fall of the Roman empire and preceded the renaissance in Europe is known to western historians as the dark ages or middle ages. What is darkest about them is our knowledge of history, for during that period writing and scholarship retreated to monasteries where monks were more concerned with preserving religious doctrines than advancing knowledge. Antecedent authority rather than inquiry was the established source of all truth. The number of teeth in the jaws of horses was debated at length, and writers cited many noted authorities for their statements. No one thought it appropriate to open the mouth of a horse and count.[1] Little was added to medical knowledge during those times.

These years of obscurity ended at various times in various parts of Europe and in various areas of knowledge. In medicine, Andreas Vesalius, who lived from 1514 to 1564, ushered in a new era of knowledge. After studying medicine in Paris, he was appointed Professor of Surgery and Anatomy at Padua in 1537. He then undertook a series of dissections of human cadavers and disputed the dogma of Galen, who had based his teachings of human anatomy on dissections of dogs and pigs. Vesalius was challenged by the church, for he found men and women both to have twelve ribs, clearly at conflict with biblical authority, which stated that God removed one of Adam's ribs to make Eve.

Alternatively, one may mark the beginning of the renaissance in medicine and science with Galileo who was born in Pisa in 1564, the year Vesalius died, and lived until 1642. Galileo studied medicine, although his contributions to the physical sciences were much greater than those he made to medicine. In fact, what stands above all other things as the contribution of Galileo is not the pendulum nor the mountains on the moon but the introduction of measurements into science. That medicine is an art is an oft repeated truism. That medicine is a science is the fact that has allowed physicians to move from the role of comforters of sick persons to healers. Interestingly, Galileo used his own pulse in timing the swings of his pendulum.

What do we know of tuberculosis in Europe between Rome and the renaissance? Very little. If savants did not count the teeth of horses, how can we be surprised that they also did not count the number of persons ill with or dying of tuberculosis. During the dark ages, people lived in small villages, largely as subsistence farmers. Their farms were ravaged periodically by invaders from the north and east. It is likely that the average agrarian European of the first millennium met no more than two to three hundred other persons in a life time. This number is similar to that noted in Chapter 1 as the minimum number needed to sustain tuberculosis in a primitive society, and Europeans between the eras of the Romans and Charlemagne may have lived more like the present Mato Grosso Indians than like the knights and ladies of legendary Camelot. At this time tuberculosis was probably sporadically distributed and not a common illness; but the scourge had not been conquered, and it would return in due time.[2]

One form of tuberculosis was well described in medieval times, and we can infer a good bit from our knowledge of it. Scrofula (or less commonly struma) was and still is the name given to tuberculosis of the lymph glands of the neck. The lymph glands in the neck below the angle of the jaw become swollen and rubbery but not tender when they are the site of tuberculosis. Experienced clinicians today have little difficulty in suspecting this diagnosis from the characteristic feel of these nodes. In earlier times, other causes of swollen lymph glands might have been confused with tuberculosis, but the chronic and relatively painless nature of scrofula makes it likely that medieval physicians were reasonably accurate in their diagnoses.

To explore the history of scrofula, we must first learn of the healing power of the royal touch. If healing of illness was accomplished by gods or God—not by physicians—and if Jesus performed His healing miracles by touching, then perhaps it was not surprising that early monarchs, who viewed their authority as of divine origin, claimed the power of healing by touching. Among those diseases for which the use of touching was most frequently employed was scrofula. Clovis of France, who

included the touching of persons with scrofula in his coronation ceremony in 496, may have been the first European monarch to touch
scrofulous persons, and for many generations his descendants claimed
to have inherited his healing power. Scrofula became known as "the
King's Evil."[3] Louis XIV is said to have touched two thousand and five
hundred persons.

Edward the Confessor, who died in 1056, was the first British ruler
to claim to be able to cure scrofula by touching. While the practice was
abandoned by his immediate successors, it was revived by Edward I,
who touched five hundred and thirty-three persons in a single month
in 1277, and reached its height in the seventeenth century. Henry VII
started the practice of giving a gold "angel"—an amulet or a gold coin
with a figure of St. Michael—to those whom he touched. The preferred
times for touching were Easter Sunday, Pentecost, and the Feast of
Michaelmas. During the reign of James I and Charles I, specific litur-
gies for use in touching were developed, some of which persisted in
prayer books until late in the nineteenth century. The ritual included
initial examination of patients by physicians to verify the diagnosis of
scrofula, prayers recited by priests, stroking of both sides of the face
with both hands by the king, hanging of a gold piece about the patient's
neck, and closing prayers and a blessing.

At the beginning of the seventeenth century, Shakespeare described
touching for scrofula in Macbeth, Act IV, scene 3,

> ". . . .strangely visited people,
> All swoln and ulcerous, pitiful to the eye,
> The mere despair of surgery, he cures;
> Hanging a golden stamp about their necks,
> Put on with holy prayers."

Samuel Johnson, one of the legendary literary figures of his time, was
born in Litchfield, England in September 1709. He was a sickly infant,
and at an early age was found to have scrofula.[4] His physician, Dr.
Swinfen, noted that his foster brother had the same disease and attributed the illness to his nurse's milk. His mother, Sarah, believed the disease had been inherited from her family, for she had several relatives
who were similarly afflicted. In 1712, when he was two and one-half,

his mother took him to London to be touched by Queen Anne, the last British monarch to practice touching regularly. Johnson later reported remembering the arduous three day coach journey. "I was sick," he reported. "One woman fondled me, the other was disgusted."

In London, the young Samuel Johnson underwent rigorous examination by the court physicians on the day before the scheduled touching to confirm his diagnosis. He then joined two hundred other scrofulous patients for the ceremony. He received a gold "touchpiece" with an impression of St. Michael the archangel on one side and of a ship in full sail on the other side. Johnson wore this medal about his neck for the rest of his life.

Samuel Johnson's scrofula was probably not benefitted by Queen Anne's royal touch. Several years later he underwent a surgical operation to open the infected lymph nodes and let them drain. The disfiguring scars from this procedure remained throughout his life. During his school years, however, the scrofula healed, and Johnson was not further troubled with tuberculosis, although he had recurrent illnesses during his later years, many of them related to heart failure. This course of scrofula was not unusual, and it may explain some of the success of the royal touch. Scrofula usually is an indolent disease, ultimately resolving spontaneously. And persons who have recovered from scrofula appear to carry some immunity to subsequent attacks of other forms of tuberculosis.

How common was scrofula in the middle ages? Apparently very common, at least late in this period. King Charles II is said to have touched ninety-two thousand people for the treatment of scrofula between 1662 and 1682, an average rate of almost ninety persons per week. At a touching ceremony held by Charles II in 1684, the crowd of persons seeking to be touched was so large that seven persons were trampled to death. Scrofula may have been more common during the reign of Charles II than at any other time in British history.

In the United States during recent years, tuberculosis of the lymph nodes has accounted for three to six percent of all tuberculosis. That is, one can multiply the number of cases of tuberculosis found in lymph nodes by fifteen to thirty and come up with the approximate number of total cases of tuberculosis. By all accounts, scrofula must have been very common in late medieval Europe. We must then assume that the enlightenment of Europe heralded by the renaissance illumined a land whose peoples were commonly afflicted with tuberculosis in all its forms.

Saint Francis of Assisi, who was born in 1182 towards the end of the dark ages but well before the dawning of the renaissance, was the son of a prosperous merchant.[5] As a youth, he fell captive in a battle between his native Assisi and the rival city of Perugia. He was imprisoned for one year. Upon release, he was ill with fever and wasting. He then began his mission among the poor, living with them, and his work revolutionized the Christian church. He died in 1226 at the age of forty-four, probably of tuberculosis, after a period of wasting illness. He was canonized by Pope Gregory IX less than two years later. By all accounts, tuberculosis at this time was widespread in prisons and among the poor. It is likely that St. Francis contracted his consumption either in prison or while living among the poor. Certainly tuberculosis was then, at the end of the dark ages, widespread among the impoverished people of Europe's cities.

As the great white plague of tuberculosis spread across Europe, it was not simply a disease of the imprisoned and the impoverished. Louis XIII of France was consumptive and died of his disease in 1643 at age forty-two; tuberculosis was also a royal malady.

The mercantile and academic communities did not escape. The Espinosa family fled from Spain to Portugal, hounded by the inquisition and forced from their homeland by the Jewish expulsion order of 1492.[6] Baptized to Christianity at sword point, they changed their name to its Portugese form, Spinoza. Somewhat more than a century later, when religious freedom was established in Holland, the Spinozas joined others in moving there. Baruch Spinoza was born in 1632 in Vloijenburg, a poor Jewish sector of Amsterdam, the third of three children of Michael Espinosa and Hana Debora Despinoza. Michael was a merchant. His wife died of tuberculosis when her youngest son was six years old; the two older siblings succumbed to this disease as children. Baruch Spinoza was an able student who pursued both Hebrew and Talmudic studies. His father prospered, and the family moved to the more affluent town of Burgwal. Baruch Spinoza, influenced by reading Decartes's writings on optics, took up lens grinding, a craft at which he became proficient. Intellectually, he became increasingly liberal and free-thinking; ultimately he was excommunicated from his Jewish synagogue. He moved to the

Hague where he prospered and became widely known throughout Europe for his writings and liberal teachings. In 1677, at age forty-four, he became ill with tuberculosis and had a rapid down-hill course that ended with his untimely death.

The postmedieval epidemic of tuberculosis in Europe probably peaked during the life time of Spinoza in the seventeenth century, riding on a tide of urbanization. John Locke, a diarist, philosopher, statesman, and well known physician of his time, reported that twenty percent of all deaths in London were due to tuberculosis in 1667.[7] Locke himself developed tuberculosis at the age of thirty-four, but he lived on to the age of seventy-two. Case rates in London during the 1600s probably reached 1,000 to 1,250 new cases each year for every 100,000 persons.[8] Tuberculosis incidences this high are rare in modern times and they occur principally in refugee camps and similar situations.

So it was that John Bunyan, one of the most widely read authors of his day, spoke not only with eloquence and vivid imagery but also with veracity in 1660 when he described tuberculosis in "The Life and Death of Mr. Badman" as, "The Captain among these Men of Death."[9]

4

The Relentless Tide

The Bay of Fundy has the highest tides in the world. Twice daily the tide surges into the narrow bay and generates a wave that moves relentlessly up the Salmon River—the tidal bore. So has the epidemic of tuberculosis, the great white plague, swept relentlessly across the inhabited earth. Humans have tried to temper its surge, and public health officials have been quick to accept credit when the tide has ebbed. Human endeavor has perhaps modified the course of the wave somewhat, and human activity—more often unintended than purposeful—has certainly modified its course. But in the end, it is not clear that humankind has been able to do other than ride the ebb and flow of this relentless tide.

Tuberculosis is not unique in its ebb and flow. All epidemic infectious diseases pursue such a pattern.[1] Measles tends to recur every two years; influenza every four. Why is this so? When measles sweeps through the children of a community or school, it afflicts nearly every child not immune from having had measles previously. At the end of this epidemic wave, essentially all of the children in the population are now immune. "Herd immunity" is the term sometimes used to describe this phenomenon. On the average, it takes about two years for a sufficient number of naive, nonimmune children to grow up into the population at risk to support another measles epidemic. In much of the world, vaccination against measles has dramatically altered this pattern, and the all too familiar cough and spots of this disease are now infrequent visitors and may soon be vanquished from the earth.[2]

Influenza occurs in a pattern of epidemics much less regular than that of measles, but immunity of the population—herd immunity—again plays an important role. Other factors being equal, it takes about four years for a sufficient number of nonimmune individuals to be present in the population to sustain a new epidemic of influenza. However, in recent years, this pattern has broken down, probably not so much because of vaccination as because people now travel so frequently that the population at risk is not simply an individual community but the whole world, and nearly every winter sees an epidemic of flu.

The influenza virus is able to change its skin like a chameleon. That is, the virus changes the antigenic structure by which our immune defense mechanisms recognize it. Whenever this occurs, a large epidemic occurs, often circling the globe. These newly altered viruses meet people who have no immunity, and the results are often devastating. Thus, in 1917 a new strain of influenza virus became established in American army training camps, was carried to Europe on troop ships, and then spread throughout the world in one of the deadliest epidemics the world has seen. Similarly, 1957 saw the United States hard hit by "Asian flu," with many deaths among its victims.

Plague and cholera are epidemic diseases that are more mysterious. Epidemics of cholera have spread across the world after cholera-free decades or centuries. The causative germ resides in contaminated water supplies. In 1854 Dr. John Snow provided an elegant demonstration of the importance of unsanitary drinking water in a neighborhood of London by removing the handle of a communal pump. Where does cholera hide between epidemics? What leads to a new wave? These questions are unanswered.

Plague is usually spread by fleas of rats, less often through the air in a pneumonic form. Waves of plague are known to have spread as epidemics across the earth since the third century before Christ, and the "Black Death" of the fourteenth century killed one-third of Europe's total population. In recent times, plague has been a rare disease, occurring only sporadically, usually in hunters or others in contact with small rodents. Yet, without obvious explanation, an outbreak of pneumonic plague occurred in India in 1994.

Do such epidemic waves occur with tuberculosis? History suggests that they may, with a time interval measured in centuries. We have seen in previous chapters that tuberculosis was common in predynastic Egypt but had largely passed as an epidemic disease by the time of Alexander's conquest. In Europe, tuberculosis was present throughout the middle ages, but it was in the seventeenth century that it reached what can only be considered astounding epidemic proportions. Richard Morton, a prominent English physician who lived from 1637 to 1698 wrote, "I cannot sufficiently advise that anyone, at least after he comes to the flower of his youth, can die without a touch of consumption."[3] Tuberculosis mortality peaked in England in 1780, early in the industrial revolution, at an incredible death rate of one thousand, one hundred and twenty for each one hundred thousand living persons each year (written by epidemiologists as 1,120/100,000/year).[4] In ordinary terms, that means that one and one-quarter percent of the entire population—all ages—died of this disease each year.

The tide of consumption receded somewhat in the eighteenth century, only to rise again in the nineteenth century before beginning a rapid decline that continued steadily until recent times[5]. At the Hôpital de Charité in Paris, two hundred and fifty out of six hundred and ninety-six—thirty-six percent—of deaths recorded in the early nineteenth century were due to tuberculosis. In London, the tuberculosis death rate was estimated to be 716/100,000/year for the first decade of the nineteenth century and 567/100,000/year for the period 1831 to 1835. Thomas Young, an English physician, estimated in 1815 that one-fourth of the population of Europe was consumptive, and in the 1830s thirty percent of deaths among English laborers were attributed to tuberculosis. Ludvig von Beethoven's mother and brother both succumbed to the disease. An exquisite example of tuberculosis of the spine is included in a collection of skeletons from the early nineteenth century at the University of Leiden.[6]

There may be no more poignant story of the ravages of nineteenth century tuberculosis than that of the talented literary Brontë family.[7] Dramatic as it is, it is not an exceptional one for that time period. Patrick Brontë brought his wife, Maria and the first five of their children to Haworth in Yorkshire in 1820 when he assumed the post of Methodist parson there. He is said to have had chronic bronchitis; more than likely, his cough was tubercular, and he probably infected his children. Prior to the move, all of the children slept in the same bedroom of their Cornwall home, the type of crowding typical of the day and favorable to the spread of airborne infections, including tuberculosis.

The youngest Brontë child, Anne, was born at Haworth, shortly after the family's move. Maria, the mother, suffered childbirth fever—

puerperal sepsis in medical terminology—and died several months later. While puerperal sepsis was frequently fatal, Maria's illness lasted longer than one would expect of childbirth fever, leading to the inevitable question of whether, in fact, she might not have had tuberculosis or some other chronic disease as a cause of her death. The Reverend Patrick Brontë soon found it difficult to care for his large, motherless family, and in 1824 he sent the four oldest girls, Maria, Elizabeth, Charlotte, and Emily to a newly opened school for the daughters of evangelical clergy at Cowan Bridge, about fifty miles from Haworth. Living conditions at this school, the model for Lowood School in Charlotte Brontë's *Jane Eyre*, were Spartan at best, and the dormitory rooms for the sixty resident girls were crowded. Epidemics of measles, typhoid fever, and typhus swept the school. Under such conditions, tuberculosis is easily spread, and the Brontë sisters may have contracted their ultimately fatal illnesses at this school rather than from their father.

Within a year in April 1825, Maria Brontë fell ill with tuberculosis. In *Jane Eyre*, Charlotte describes the illness of Jane's friend Helen Burns at Lowood. "Helen was ill at present . . . She was not, I was told, in the hospital portion of the house with the fever patients, for her complaint was consumption, not typhus; and by consumption I, in my ignorance, understood something mild, which time and care would be sure to alleviate." This passage probably describes the illness of Charlotte's younger sister, Maria. Maria returned home to Haworth from Cowan Bridge, to die on May 6, 1825 at the age of twelve, the first of these remarkable six children to fall victim to consumption. Charlotte and Emily were then withdrawn from the harsh environment of Cowan Bridge, and Elizabeth followed her sister to die of tuberculosis on June 1, 1825 at the age of eleven.

In 1846, Charlotte Brontë began writing *Jane Eyre*, one of the most popular novels of its time and an enduring classic. Two years later, death from tuberculosis visited the Brontë family again, claiming the only son, Branwell, on September 24 and Emily on December 19. In a letter to a friend written shortly after Emily's death, Charlotte said of her sister's illness and death, ". . . .the elements bring her no more suffering—their severity cannot reach her grave—her fever is quieted, her restlessness soothed, her deep hollow cough is hushed forever; we do not hear it in the night nor listen for it in the morning; we have not the

conflict of the strangely strong spirit and the fragile frame before us. . . ."[8]
In January 1849, two weeks after Emily's death, Anne Brontë, the young-
est child of this family, was found to have tuberculosis. She died on
May 28 at the age of twenty-nine after a wasting course.

Charlotte Brontë lived to the age thirty-eight; she died in 1855 one
year after her marriage. A portrait of the already famous author done in
chalk by George Richard five years before her death now hangs in the
National Portrait Gallery in London. It shows a woman with a thin
face, perhaps chronically ill. Charlotte died of a wasting illness that was
at least complicated by severe nausea and vomiting associated with pregnancy. While she suffered much ill health during her pregnancy, it was
probably tuberculosis that brought her down to the grave. The Reverend Patrick Brontë lived on to the age of eighty-five.

In 1882, Robert Koch, the discoverer of the tubercle bacillus and one
of the greatest scientists of his time, introduced his classic paper on the
cause of tuberculosis by noting its importance as a cause of death in
Europe of his day. "If the number of victims which a disease claims is
the measure of its significance, then all diseases, particularly the most
dreaded infectious diseases, such as bubonic plague, Asiatic cholera,
etc., must rank far behind tuberculosis. Statistics teach that one-seventh of all human beings die of tuberculosis, and that, if one considers
only the productive middle-age groups, tuberculosis carries away one-
third and often more of these."[9]

With tuberculosis now well established among all classes of Europe's
citizens and with many of the continent's leading intellectuals and artists afflicted, the disease became romanticized, and the thin, pale face of
the consumptive was considered beautiful. The romantic and acclaimed
poet Lord Byron is said to have told a friend, "I should like to die of a
consumption. . . .because the ladies would say, 'look at that poor Byron.
How interesting he looks in dying.'" A mid nineteenth century paint-
ing by William Morris, depicting the legendary Guinevere, King Arthur's
queen, shows a thin, pale face, the concept of beauty of the romantic
age again encompassing the wasting of consumption.

Nowhere is the wan visage of consumption better portrayed than in
the statue of Edward Livingston Trudeau sculpted by Gutzon Borglum
(Figure 4.1). The famous physician, whose story is recounted in Chapter 21, developed tuberculosis in 1873, less than two decades after Char-

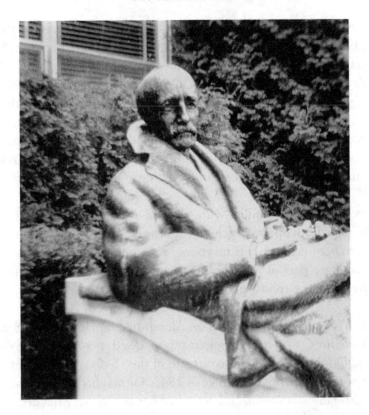

Figure 4.1. Edward Livingston Trudeau sculpted as a patient with tuberculosis by Gutzon Borglum. The statue stands on the grounds of the Trudeau Institute in Saranac Lake. Photograph by the author.

lotte Brontë died of tuberculosis and William Morris painted a consumptive Guinevere.

Oliver Twist, the juvenile protagonist of Charles Dickens' famous 1838 novel, was born in a workhouse. His mother is romantically described by Dickens in a passage that reads, "the pale face of a young woman was raised feebly from the pillow; and a faint voice imperfectly articulated the words, 'Let me see the child, and die.'" Her death at the beginning of the novel leaves Oliver an orphan. Dickens does not offer a cause of death for this pale woman; perhaps he might have chosen tuberculosis, for it was rampant in English workhouses of the time. In 1844, a survey in an English workhouse found that all of seventy-eight boys and ninety-one of ninety-four girls showed signs of the disease.

Harvard University was founded in 1636. In 1639 it was named for John Harvard in gratitude for his bequest of money and books. In 1884 Daniel Chester French completed the statue of John Harvard which stands today in the Harvard Yard. No portraits of Harvard existed, and French went to the Harvard library to learn what he could of the appearance of his subject. French reported of John Harvard that "it is recorded that he died at the age of about thirty of consumption and that gave a clue to the sort of physique that he had. It is fair to assume that his face would be delicate in modeling and sensitive in expression. . . ."[10]

Opera lovers are familiar with Violetta of *La Traviata* and Mimi of *La Bohème*. Both operas conclude with the heroines dying of tuberculosis. Both heroines are beautiful young women, and their thin, consumptive faces are part of their beauty (modern opera goers may have to forgive the more robust physiognomies of many contemporary sopranos).

Verdi's *La Traviata* was based on Alexandre Dumas' (fils) 1848 novel *La Dame aux Camélias,* and Violetta was modeled after Alphonsine Plessis (Marie Duplessis), a famous courtesan of the 1840s who died of tuberculosis at the age of twenty-three in 1847. Dumas had a romantic affair with this famous woman, and described her as "tall, very slender, black-haired, and with a pink-and-white complexion." As she approaches death in Act 4 of the opera, Violetta sings, "Ah, how my face is altered. . . . Farewell happy dreams of the time that has fled! My cheeks's blooming roses are faded and dead."[11]

Puccini's *La Bohème* premiered in Turin in 1896 with the young Arturo Toscannini conducting. At that time, tuberculosis was beginning to wane in Europe, although it still was very familiar to most of the audience. The initial reception of this opera, although favorable, hardly was clamorous and did not foretell the immense popularity the work was soon to achieve. *La Bohème* was based on Henri Murger's autobiographical novel *Scenes de la Vie de Bohème*; it is set in about 1830. Like Violetta, Mimi notes her pallor as her death approaches. She asks Rudolfo, "Am I still beautiful?"

"As beautiful as a dawn," he replies.

"You employed the wrong figure, you meant to say beautiful as a sunset."[12]

Tides are not confined to the Bay of Fundy; they circle the earth. So also, tuberculosis was not confined to Europe, and it spread like a tide across the globe, often transported by diseased Europeans during their explorations, conquests, and colonizations.

Half of the Pilgrims who reached Plymouth, Massachusetts in 1620 died during their first winter. Although some authors suggest that tuberculosis was among the causes of death that swept through that colony, documentation to support this assertion is lacking. In fact, no physicians accompanied the colonists who sailed on the Mayflower. Some contemporary observers of New England at the end of the seventeenth century and early in the eighteenth century felt that its brisk climate and pure air protected its residents from consumption, noting that it was much less commonly seen than in Europe. However, Cotton Mather, whose wife died of tuberculosis in 1702 and who probably had the disease himself, and others writing at the same time described a number of clear-cut cases of tuberculosis. By the time of the Revolutionary War, tuberculosis was well established, accounting for about one in every five to seven deaths in New England. By the beginning of the nineteenth century, tuberculosis was recorded as the cause of twenty-three percent of deaths in Salem, Massachusetts, twenty-seven percent of deaths in Brookline, Massachusetts, and twenty to twenty-five percent of deaths in New York City.[13] Henry David Thoreau, who retreated to Walden Pond primarily in hopes of achieving a cure, and Nathaniel Hawthorne both died of tuberculosis. Ralph Waldo Emerson suffered from the disease, but survived it.

We have seen in Chapter 1 that tuberculosis was present in the indigenous populations of North America. In fact, a burial mound near Cincinnati, Ohio dated at 1275 yielded skeletal remains of one hundred and ninety persons, six of whom had bony changes characteristic of tuberculosis.[14] An Iroquoian ossuary near Toronto, Ontario dated to 1490 yielded evidence of tuberculosis in twenty-four of four hundred and fifty-seven skeletons.[15] But this disease was not common among most groups of North American Indians at the time the colonialists pushed west. Benjamin Rush, an eminent statesman, signer of the Declaration of Independence, and physician of the eighteenth century, reported that tuberculosis was unknown in the Indian population.[16] Certainly it is true that many of the previously uninfected native American people of that time were highly susceptible to this disease as well as others brought to them by their colonialist conquerors, and death rates among Indians soon soared. Pere Jacques Marquette, who explored much of the upper Great Lakes and left his name on a city in Michigan and a street in Minneapolis, died of tuberculosis in 1674.

Tuberculosis appears to have been rare or unknown among native Americans of the arctic prior their contact with early explorers.[17] Captain W.E. Parry, who explored the Canadian Arctic between 1818 and 1825 found the Eskimos to be largely free of most of the infectious diseases he knew, as did other early explorers. Parry did describe one native youth as "consumptive-looking," but of greater import was the fact that one of his sailors died from consumption during his second voyage. Then came the gold rush of the late nineteenth century. Tuberculosis was introduced into the coastal towns and spread explosively.

The first systematic survey of the tuberculosis problem among Alaskan natives was conducted between 1948 and 1951. At that time an astounding ninety percent of five and six year-old children living in the Yukon and Kuskokwim River delta area were found to be infected with tubercle bacilli, and thirty percent of adults had chest radiographic evidence of clinical tuberculosis. There are no other recorded rates of infection and disease this high in any population. Since then, dramatic decreases in tuberculosis have occurred in this population. A major control program mounted by the United States Public Health Service and dramatically improved living conditions probably share the credit for this success story.

Tuberculosis spread not only to North America but across the world in the wake of European colonizers. The accounts of early sea captains indicate that it was rare or nonexistent in South and West Africa, but this situation changed with European exploration. James Bruce and Cecil Rhodes probably had tuberculosis. Early records make scant mention of tuberculosis—called "tap-dikh" by Punjabis—but by 1900 it was responsible for approximately ten percent of deaths recorded in Indian cities.[18] Nor did the emerging nations of South America escape consumption, the white plague. Simon Bolivar, the Great Libertador, was afflicted.

The poignant story of the Pitcairn Islanders epitomizes the effects of tuberculosis upon populations that are naive to it.[19] When Fletcher Christian and his comrades seized H.M.S. Bounty from Captain Bligh in their famous mutiny of April 28, 1789, they sought an island home remote from the reaches of British maritime law. They found their retreat on uninhabited and idyllic, tropical Pitcairn Island, and on January 23, 1790 the band of British seamen and their Tahitian families—twenty-eight persons—burned the Bounty on the rocky shore of their new home, thus cutting all connection with the outer world. They prospered and were healthy, and by 1831 the population of Pitcairn Island had grown to eighty-six. In that year, they were convinced to return to Tahiti, where for the first time they met many infectious diseases, including tuberculosis. Unhappy in Tahiti, they returned to Pitcairn Island after only six months, but epidemic disease was unstoppable. Within six months the Pitcairn Islanders numbered only seventeen persons. In 1838 they were visited by Captain Elliott of H.M. Sloop Fly, who noted consumption and scrofula among the islanders. Records kept on the island document that of one hundred and fourteen deaths recorded during the seven decades from 1864 to 1934 twelve—one in ten—were due to tuberculosis. Only accidents took a higher toll.

Tides ebb, and so have epidemics of tuberculosis. In the words of one noted student of tuberculosis, "Disease cycles may be very long, they may even, although probably rarely, take centuries to finish their course, but in the end the wave *must* finish its rise, and inevitably fall, and the particular parasite as a group infection must, temporarily at least, cease to be a menace to its particular group host."[20] The turning point in England appears to have come about 1850. It was perhaps a little earlier in New England. Tuberculosis receded dramatically, at a rate that makes one ready to abandon the metaphor of a tide, and the decline has continued so steadily that many thoughtful students of tuberculosis have felt impelled to ask how and why.

Thomas McKeown, a distinguished population scientist, was among the first to address these questions thoughtfully. Death registration began in England and Wales in 1838. McKeown compared deaths rates in the sixth and tenth decades of nineteenth century Britain.[21] Overall, mortality fell from 2,121/100,000/year to 1,812/100,000/year, a fourteen and one-half percent decrease in forty years. Mortality from tuberculosis of all forms declined from 348/100,000/year to 202/100,000/year, nearly a forty-three percent decline. The decrease in tuberculosis mortality began approximately thirty years before similar decreases in deaths from other infectious diseases and accounted for almost half of the total decrease in mortality during the half century reviewed.

McKeown carefully considered various possible explanations for the rapid decline in tuberculosis mortality. Genetic changes in the people of Britain seemed to him an unlikely explanation, because one would expect such changes to need many generations to develop and to have a major impact. Were it possible for people to have evolved into more resistant beings within such a period of time, one would have expected similar resistance to have developed among many third world populations during the past century or more when they have encountered this disease, and that has not happened.

McKeown notes that no effective therapy for tuberculosis, which might have made patients less infectious, was introduced during this time. Nor did standards of housing improve; during this time period the number of persons in each dwelling fell no more than from five and two-thirds to five and one-third. After careful consideration, McKeown concluded that better nutrition was the most likely explanation. He noted that food production increased rapidly during this time. So also did the population of consumers, but from 1870 forward the increase in food production exceeded population growth. Concomitantly, the industrial revolution brought an increase in real wages, allowing for purchase of more and better food.[22] Modern studies have shown that individuals who are ten percent underweight are more than three times as likely to develop tuberculosis as those who are similarly overweight.[23]

Leonard Wilson, who relied heavily on data collected by Arthur Newsholme, rejected McKeown's hypothesis.[24] He noted that during the time in question, great strides were made in the diagnosis of tuberculosis and that the practice on confining consumptives to institutions—whether hospitals or workhouses—began. Thus, he concludes, the transmission of tubercle bacilli to uninfected persons was probably impeded. While not embracing Wilson's explanation, other contemporary epidemiologists have considered this factor a possible contributor. However, the decline in tuberculosis occurred at a time when the number of infectious persons actually confined to institutions comprised only a small fraction of those who were contagious.[25] Moreover, there is substantial evidence that almost all persons who will be infected by an individual with tuberculosis are infected before the diagnosis is made, even with much more advanced case finding programs than existed in nineteenth century Britain. A landmark study in India found that no more tuberculosis occurred among the children of hospitalized tuberculosis patients than among the children to patients treated in their homes.[26] These children were infected before a diagnosis of tuberculosis was made in their parents.

Did "herd immunity" cause the nineteenth century European and North American epidemic wave of tuberculosis to recede? E.R.N. Grigg carefully analyzed European mortality data and the evidence for waves of tuberculosis over history and concluded that they could "only be fully explained by the natural selection of individuals which were (and/or had become) insusceptible to the disease."[27] In more contemporary times, this view has been embraced by Joseph Bates and William Stead,[28] both of whom have contributed enormously to many areas of our understanding of tuberculosis. However, as noted above, the rapid decline of tuberculosis makes genetic selection an unlikely factor of major importance.

Finally, as if to confound whatever analysis one wishes to make, France has refused to play the game! Despite general similarities with Britain in all of the candidates for causes of the decline of tuberculosis, mortality in that country did not begin to fall until after the first World War.[29]

What can we conclude? Certainly there have been waves of tuberculosis occurring in major populations of the earth over the span of history. Figure 4.2 schematically presents this concept for those parts of history and of the globe for which we can make reasonable inferences. There may well have been other waves of this disease in populations about which we know less. And there may have been undocumented waves at earlier times. What does seem to be true is that the tide of tuberculosis rises and falls just as certainly as the tidal does bore in the Salmon River at the head of the Bay of Fundy.

While those of us who live in Europe and North America can smugly review our history and document the decline of tuberculosis in our midst to levels that clearly indicate that the epidemic wave has past, most of the world's people live in places where tuberculosis remains among the most important of health problems. Case rates in developing countries are ten to twenty-fold those in technologically advanced countries. The tuberculosis tide has crested in much of the world, even

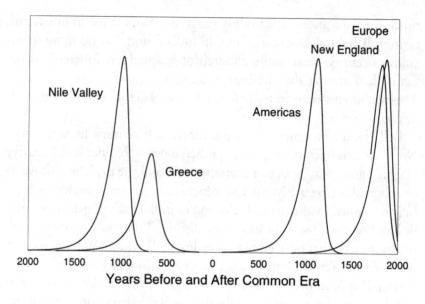

Figure 4.2. Schematic representation of five epidemic waves of tuberculosis in various locations and at various times in history. Although each wave spans centuries, the peak incidence of disease probably only lasts for a few decades. It is likely that, in general, the decline of receding waves has been somewhat more rapid than the onset of new waves, although no others probably ebbed with the speed of that in western Europe and North America in the second half of the nineteenth century.

in impoverished developing countries, but as we will see in Chapter 17, the advent of AIDS threatens to rewrite the scenario of past epochs and bring on new surges of epidemic tuberculosis. Nor can we ignore the plight of our poorer neighbors, for travelers and immigrants carry this disease with them as they move to richer parts of the world. If we are to remain free of tuberculosis, ultimately this great plague will have to be controlled on all of the surface of the globe.

5

The Hope for Eradication

In November 1962 Eleanor Roosevelt died at the age of seventy-five of a rare form of disseminated tuberculosis.[1] She probably suffered an episode of pleurisy as a young woman while working as a volunteer at a settlement house in New York City. Pleurisy was common in young people at that time, and although it often marked initial infection with the tubercle bacillus, it was usually considered an unimportant illness. Eleanor Roosevelt recovered from her bout of pleurisy, as did almost all who acquired tuberculosis of this form. Some six years later, while in France, she apparently developed active tuberculosis of her lungs, but she recovered from this illness as well and lived a long and vigorous life of robust good health. Tuberculosis did not revisit her during those many years. Only in her last two years did her health begin to fail, and she was thought to have aplastic anemia. She was treated with Cortisone, the appropriate medicine for aplastic anemia but also a drug that increases the likelihood of spread of tuberculous infection. And a spread of tuberculosis did occur, almost certainly from the long-dormant germs that had originally infected her more than fifty years previously. All parts of her body were affected. Her diagnosis was made when tuberculosis germs were isolated from her bone marrow, too late for treatment to benefit her.

There is a lesson in the story of Eleanor Roosevelt's illness. She recovered from her initial bouts, with this plague, lived a long and vigorous life, and then succumbed to tuberculosis in late life. The lesson of her story has major importance for tuberculosis control programs; it was first understood by Wade Hampton Frost.

Wade Hampton Frost was born on March 3, 1880 in Marshall, Virginia into a family of three generations of physicians.[2] His primary schooling at home was followed by a military academy and then the University of Virginia for both undergraduate and medical education.

After receiving his M.D. degree in 1903 and completing an internship in Norfolk, Virginia in 1905, Frost entered the United States Public Health Service, in which he served for the next fourteen years. His initial assignments included investigations of outbreaks of yellow fever, typhus, typhoid, and polio.

In 1917 Frost developed pulmonary tuberculosis. Relieved of duty because of his illness, he went to a sanatorium near Asheville, North Carolina for six months, returning at the end of this period to a further six months of light duty. His doctors found his tuberculosis to be arrested then, and he remained free of disease throughout the remainder of his life.

In 1919 the Johns Hopkins School of Hygiene and Public Health was established. Dr. William Welch recognized Frost as a promising star in the new and rapidly developing firmament of epidemiology. Welch secured a Public Health Service assignment for Frost detailing him to the Johns Hopkins faculty. There he remained for the rest of his extraordinarily productive career, rising to be a distinguished professor. He was one of the founders of the American Public Health Association in 1929. During the last ten years of his life Frost became concerned with the techniques of studying families over a period of time. He applied his methods to the study of tuberculosis, and he contributed enormously to our understanding of the epidemiology of that disease.

Eleanor Roosevelt was born in 1884; Wade Hampton Frost in 1880. They were contemporaries. How can it be that Eleanor Roosevelt's tuberculous infection could heal and then remain dormant for more than five decades only to reactivate and kill her? Why did Frost develop his tuberculosis at age thirty-seven and live the rest of his life free of disease after it became arrested? And what do Roosevelt's and Frost's stories imply for the course of the epidemic of tuberculosis in the community at large? Some of the answers to these questions will be addressed in later chapters of this book. For now, as we try to understand the role of tuberculosis in the lives of these two exceptional people, we must examine the disease in relation to the age of its victims and to the prevalence of tuberculosis in their era. In doing so, we will gain further understanding of this plague and the lessons taught by the illnesses of individuals such as Roosevelt and Frost. The answers to our questions come from the studies of Wade Hampton Frost himself.

We saw in the previous chapter that the tuberculosis epidemic crested in England early in the nineteenth century and then began to recede. In North America, the earliest estimates of mortality come from records in New England and Eastern Seaboard cities at the middle of the nine-teenth century. They suggest tuberculosis death rates of approximately 300/100,000/year at that time.[3] Subsequent records show a steady and progressive decline. At the same time that tuberculosis was decreasing, a shift in the nature of the disease became apparent. Increasingly tuber-culosis was becoming a disease of the elderly rather than of the young adults whom most doctors had come to recognize as its most frequent victims. Wade Hampton Frost put these two observations together to obtain new insights into this disease.

In a landmark paper published posthumously,[4] Frost noted that if people were divided into groups or cohorts according to the time at which they were born, then within each group regardless of the year of birth, tuberculosis was most frequent during the young adult years. However, as decades passed, the portion of the overall tuberculosis bur-den in the population represented by young adults declined and the portion attributable to older individuals increased.

In all populations of persons infected with tubercle bacilli, tubercu-losis tends to hit young adults the hardest, with most of the disease occurring in that age group. That fact was well understood by physi-cians in Frost's era. However, in reviewing public health data from Mas-sachusetts, Frost noted that a group of individuals born in 1880, for example, had a high peak of tuberculosis in 1900, when they were twenty years old. In 1950, when they were seventy years old, they would have a much lower peak. However, twenty-year-olds in 1950, who were born in 1930, were exposed to much less chance of tuberculous infection. The high age-twenty peak in this second cohort occurring in the year 1950 was actually lower than the low seventy year old level for the highly infected group born in 1880. Thus, the rapidly waning tuberculosis epidemic inevitably meant that more tuberculosis would be seen in eld-erly patients, like Eleanor Roosevelt, and fewer in younger persons, like Frost himself and the Brontës. Tuberculosis was becoming a senior citizen's disease. To Frost this meant that, "the balance is already against the survival of the tubercle bacillus; and we may reasonably expect that the disease will eventually be eradicated."[5]

As the twentieth century advanced, tuberculosis also began to recede—albeit slowly—from the shores and lands of the vast and primitive reaches of the developing world. For the most part, developing countries do not have reliable vital and public health statistics available for analysis. However, Karel Styblo and his colleagues at the Tuberculosis Surveillance Research Unit in the Netherlands developed methods for determining the risk of tuberculous infection using the tuberculin skin test, of which we shall learn more in Chapter 13. In 1978, they reported that tuberculosis was not only decreasing dramatically in North America and Europe but that it was also declining—albeit less dramatically—in several countries they surveyed in Africa.[6] In 1976, Anthony Lowell at the United States Public Health Service Center for Disease Control assembled available world data and projected continuously declining tuberculosis incidence for all regions of the world.[7] He noted wryly, however, that the global tuberculosis case burden would increase, because populations were increasing more rapidly than the number of cases per unit of population were decreasing.

Success begets success, and it is clear in retrospect that any program mounted in North America or Europe to control tuberculosis in the early and mid portion of the twentieth century was bound to succeed. And so it happened. In 1892 a tuberculosis association was organized in Philadelphia, the first voluntary health agency of any type in the United States. In 1904, Einar Holboell, a Danish postal clerk suggested the sale of a special stamp to raise money for the benefit of tuberculous children. The idea captured the imagination of King Christian, and it then spread from Denmark to other Scandinavian counties. In the United States, Emily Bissell took up the cause and designed a one cent Christmas seal showing a holly wreath and the words "Merry Christmas" in order to raise money to support a tuberculosis hospital in Delaware. She persuaded postal officials to permit her to sell her seals in the lobby of a post office in Wilmington, Delaware. Sales went slowly at first. Then, under the slogan "Stamp Out Tuberculosis," the Philadelphia newspaper *The North American* began publicizing Emily Bissell's efforts. President Teddy Roosevelt endorsed the new seals. In excess of three thousand dollars—ten times the original goal and a lot of money in those days—was raised in this first Christmas seal campaign in America. Under sponsorship of the American Red Cross, subsequent annual campaigns were held, each raising more money. America's aviation hero, Charles Lindberg, signed on and joined Emily Bissell in her campaign. In 1920, the National Tuberculosis Association took over Christmas seals from the Red Cross, and the familiar double-barred cross was introduced.[8] Christmas seals became a familiar part of the December holiday season. Figure 5.1 shows President John F. Kennedy accepting sheets of Christmas seals from a young girl from Cleveland who had recovered from tuberculosis.

Health departments rallied to the cause, and public campaigns against coughing and spitting in public were instituted throughout the country. But it was the mass chest radiology campaigns, with their highly visible trucks and buses, that came to epitomize America's crusade against tuberculosis. William Conrad Roentgen discovered Xrays in 1895. He was recognized for this work by the award of the first Nobel Prize in Physics in 1901; Koch did not receive his Nobel Prize in Medicine for his discovery of the tubercle bacillus until 1905. One year after Roentgen, in 1896, Thomas Alva Edison invented the Xray fluoroscope. By the 1920s the utility of chest radiographic examinations for the diagnosis of tuberculosis had become recognized. During World War II, the need for rapid examination of thousands of military recruits fostered the development of equipment for rapid, mass chest radiologic examinations; Edison's fluoroscope provided the basis for this development. In 1947 the newly established Division of Tuberculosis Control of the United States Public Health Service began to give grants to states and cities for tuberculosis control programs, and mobile chest radiology teams became a major tool of these programs. Millions of Americans were screened for tuberculosis.[9]

In Cuyahoga County, Ohio (greater metropolitan Cleveland), nearly seven hundred thousand persons, representing sixty-five percent of the adult population, received chest Xray examinations during a six month campaign in 1949. In 1951 and 1953, U.S. postal cancellations carried messages urging everyone to have a chest radiogram. However, as the mass chest radiology campaign moved from youthful enthusiasm to midlife self-inspection, it became apparent that the success of this technique was to be limited. In fact, the major utilizers of the survey buses parked on neighborhood street corners were patients with tuberculosis already known to the public health system, already on treatment, and

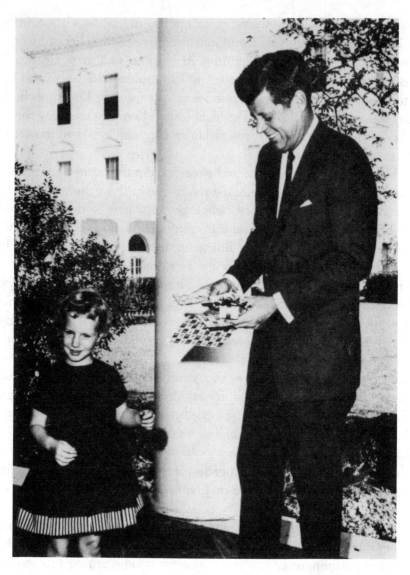

Figure 5.1. A four year-old girl from Cleveland presenting Christmas seals to President John F. Kennedy. Three years earlier this girl, then an infant of one, developed tuberculosis, which she and her brother contracted from their mother. All three of them were treated successfully and cured. Now four decades later, the young girl is healthy, married, the mother of two children, and teaching school full time. Photograph courtesy of the American Lung Association of Northern Ohio.[10]

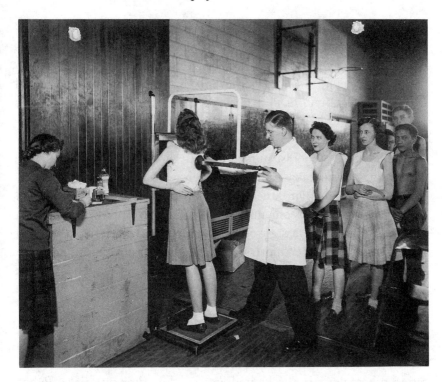

Figure 5.2. Chest radiographs being taken in the gymnasium of a Wilmington, Delaware High School in 1943 as part of a tuberculosis case finding campaign. Photograph courtesy of the American Lung Association.

anxious to check up on their doctors. Moreover, as tuberculosis continued its decline, the yield of newly discovered cases also declined. In 1966, a chest radiographic survey of more than twenty-five hundred New York City taxi drivers, a group thought to have a great deal of tuberculosis, found only one case of advanced tuberculosis. And so the Xray buses disappeared to be replaced by centralized clinics.

During World War II, tuberculosis swept like a wild fire storm through certain war-torn populations. Not only in concentration camps but also in war-ravaged civilian populations did this captain of death reap his grim harvest. Following the war in 1946 and 1947, under the energetic leadership of Johannes Holm, the Danish Red Cross began a campaign of tuberculosis control in Europe.[11] Vaccination with BCG, a vaccine against tuberculosis that was developed decades earlier and that is discussed in

Chapter 15, was the principal public health tool employed. The campaign also included screening for tuberculous infection, and this screening reached more than thirteen million persons. The remarkable international cooperation achieved during this campaign became a model for future collaborations in many areas of public interest.

As tuberculosis became a less frequent visitor to Americans and Europeans, it became more often seen as the cause of outbreaks of disease or microepidemics. Schools, nursing homes, homeless shelters were the sites of these outbreaks—all places where susceptible persons congregated. The closed environments of navy ships provided fertile ground for several such microepidemics. In 1959, an electrician serving on a picket destroyer with a crew of two hundred and thirty-six developed active pulmonary tuberculosis with a cough and tuberculosis germs in his sputum.[12] His infection exposed his shipmates, and by the time the small epidemic had run its course over the ensuing eighteen months, three additional sailors had developed active tuberculosis. Thirty-three other seamen became infected but did not develop clinical disease.

In 1959, the National Tuberculosis Association and the Public Health Service jointly sponsored a conference to consider the prospects for eradicating tuberculosis in the United States.[13] The time was right. Public health statistics demonstrated a continued decline in the disease in North America, and a further decrease to half the current levels was anticipated over the coming decade. Effective drug treatment had been introduced within the prior decade, and this treatment was being applied not only to cases of active disease but also to individuals who were infected but not yet diseased in a form of prophylaxis. When the conferees met, they were filled with optimism, hope, and excitement.

Twenty conferees—the elite of American tuberculosis and public health experts—assembled at Arden House in Harriman, New York, on November 29, 1959. Included among them were Esmond R. Long, Director of the Phipps Institute of the University of Pennsylvania and the acknowledged dean of tuberculosis research; Rene DuBos of the Rockefeller Institute, whose studies of the tuberculosis germ had set the stage for much the discovery of effective drug treatment; Alexander D. Langmuir, Chief of the Epidemiology Branch of the Communicable Disease Center of the US Public Health Service; and Walsh McDermott, Chairman of the Department of Public Health and Preventive Medicine at Cornell University Medical Center and Editor of *The American Review of Respiratory Diseases,* the leading medical journal publishing research on tuberculosis. The conferees were a group of carefully selected tuberculosis research and public health experts.

As its major recommendation, the conference recommended "a program for the widespread application of chemotherapy [drug treatment, TMD] as a public health measure for the elimination of tuberculosis in the United States." The conference recommendations skirted the issue of what was meant by "elimination of tuberculosis." Reduction to some very low level of new cases was clearly intended, but what this low level should be was not specified. However, the gauntlet was clearly on the tourney field. The challenge was there, and people rose to meet it. With the recommendations of the Arden House conference widely circulated, health departments, clinics, and lung associations throughout the country took up the banner. Success was imminent, and progress was made. In 1987 the Secretary of the Department of Health and Human Services established an Advisory Committee for the Elimination of Tuberculosis.[14] This time, elimination was clearly defined. The goal was a case rate of fewer than one new case of tuberculosis each year for each million people in the United States by the year 2010. The goal seemed achievable. The methods to be employed by and large reprised those enumerated at Arden House.

Victory was in sight. The final push was on.

6

The Failed Conquest

What went wrong?

In 1953, a national case reporting system for tuberculosis was established for the United States. As the reports rolled in, they documented that year after year, without exception fewer new cases of tuberculosis occurred in the United States each year than in the preceding year. In 1953, eighty-four thousand new cases were reported, in 1963 fifty-four thousand, in 1973 thirty-one thousand, and in 1983 twenty-two thousand. In 1985, the number was again twenty-two thousand. Then, in 1986, for the first time in the history of American tuberculosis case reporting an increase occurred. There were twenty-three thousand new cases. In 1987, 1988, and 1989 the numbers were similar, and in each subsequent year more tuberculosis until 1993, when the rising tide finally abated. Figure 6.1 illustrates the steadily declining trend in tuberculosis case rates beginning in 1953 when the first data are available and the reversal of this trend in the mid 1980s. While this reversal may not look impressive on the scale of the figure, it is unique in the history of the United States. Moreover, by 1993, some sixty thousand persons had developed disease who would not have done so had the well established trend of declining tuberculosis incidence continued.

What went wrong? *The New York Times* headlined the lead story on the first page of its edition of July 15, 1990, "Tuberculosis Germ Resurges as Peril to Public Health. Highest Threat in Cities. Re-emergence Borne on Tide of AIDS, Homelessness, Drugs and Alcohol Abuse." *The New York Times* had it right, or almost right. Add in immigration from high prevalence areas of the world and add in a collapse of public health control measures in some parts of the United States, including New York City, and one has a list of the major factors responsible for the

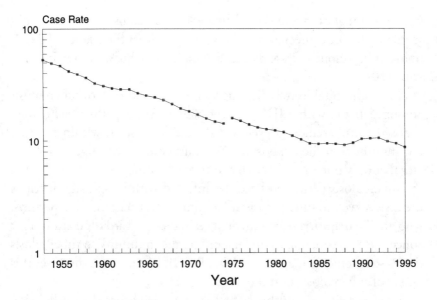

Figure 6.1. Tuberculosis case rates as the number of new cases per 100,000 population for 1955 through 1995. The apparent break in 1975 is due to a change in the criteria used for reporting cases. Over the period of four decades, the decline in tuberculosis is constant and uninterrupted until the mid 1980s. At that time, tuberculosis incidence leveled and then slowly increased, for the first time in documented US history. Beginning in 1993, tuberculosis incidence appears to be declining again in parallel with its previously established rate of decline. Data from annual reports of the Division of Tuberculosis Elimination, Centers for Disease Control and Prevention, Atlanta, GA.

unprecedented and unexpected reversal of medical history that made tuberculosis once again a feared and all too common plague in America.

AIDS was described in the United States in 1982. Soon thereafter, in 1986, doctors in Newark, New Jersey reported that many of their AIDS patients also had tuberculosis,[1] and it rapidly became evident that tuberculosis was a major infectious complication of AIDS. The cause of AIDS is the human immunodeficiency virus—HIV, and HIV attacks first and foremost precisely those cells of the immune system responsible for protection against tuberculosis. Soon, doctors in New York

City noted that drug addicts infected with tuberculosis germs who sub-sequently became infected with HIV had ten times the chance of developing tuberculous disease as did drug addicts who were not infected with HIV.[2]

A small hospital in Italy was the scene of an outbreak of tuberculosis among patients with AIDS. Nearly half of AIDS patients who were exposed to tuberculosis developed disease, almost all within the first few months after their exposure.[3] We must contrast this figure with the fact that only one in every twelve to twenty normal persons who meets the tuberculosis germ and becomes infected with it, actually develops the disease we call tuberculosis at any time. The other infected persons, who are the majority, have sufficient resistance to ward off disease. This concept is fundamental to understanding the immunity to tuberculosis that is so severely damaged by AIDS. Part III of this book discusses this aspect of tuberculosis in more detail.

Early in 1991, an outbreak of tuberculosis occurred in a housing facility for persons infected with HIV in San Francisco.[4] An AIDS pa-tient with infectious tuberculosis came to live there. The facility had thirty-two private bedrooms, but shared bathrooms and a shared kitchen and common rooms on the first floor. Over the next four months, eleven residents developed tuberculosis, and four other residents became in-fected but did not develop disease. Using DNA fingerprinting, the fo-rensic technique so much publicized for its ability to trace blood stains to their source in criminal investigations, scientists in California were able to demonstrate that all of the cases of tuberculosis came from the same source—the newly arrived tuberculous patient.

We know that tuberculosis is an infectious disease, and we know that this disease spreads from one person to the next. But never prior to the AIDS epidemic have the attack rates following exposure been as high as they are in HIV-infected persons.

Nowhere in the world has the resurgence of tuberculosis been as fright-eningly dramatic as in the crowded slums of New York City. In ten short years from 1979, when it reached its lowest point, to 1989, the tuberculosis case rate in central Harlem more than tripled.[5] Who were these people in Harlem who became the victims of tuberculosis. Forty percent were HIV-infected; sixty percent were not. Eighty-two percent were unemployed and sixty-eight percent were homeless or unstably housed. More than half were alcoholics and more than half intravenous drug users. These people were and still are the neglected people of our inner cities, many of whom we once housed in institutions but have now turned out onto the streets. They are our tired, our poor, our huddled masses. As inscribed on the Statue of Liberty, our immigrants who fit this description are "yearning to breathe free." As today's tired and poor walking the streets of our modern cities, they breathe not only freely but contagiously, expiring tuberculosis germs, a public health hazard to all.

Nearly one-third of the persons who develop tuberculosis in the United States were born in other lands. In South Florida, they have come from Haiti; in Texas, from Mexico; in California, from the Philippines. All of those countries have tuberculosis case rates many fold those in America, and immigrants from those countries bring their tuberculosis risk with them. Selected data on tuberculosis among foreign-born persons in the United States by country of origin are presented in Table 6.1. Mexicans bring more tuberculosis to this country than any other group, for there are many immigrants from that country. The actual case rates of tuberculosis are highest in persons from countries in Southeast Asia, but fewer of them come to North America. Moreover, it is now clear that these recent arrivals continue to transmit this disease within their new communities, principally to their own children.

A strain of tubercle bacilli brought from Korea swept through an American high school, infecting as many as fifty students. Worse, the strain was resistant to the drug usually used to treat tuberculous infection.[6] Modern DNA fingerprinting techniques have demonstrated that three Dutch tuberculosis patients acquired their infections while residing or traveling in Ethiopia or Tunisia.[7]

A frightening aspect of the tuberculosis outbreak in the United States and particularly in New York City is the emergence of strains of tuberculosis germs that are resistant to most or all of the drugs available for treatment of tuberculosis. The multidrug-resistant—"MDR"—strains first emerged among AIDS patients in New York and then spread rapidly through the poorly ventilated prisons of New York State. They have proven to be lethal in AIDS patients. Immunologically normal persons can also be infected—and many doctors, nurses, and prison employees have been—but they handle the germ with the same sort of resistance

Table 6.1
Tuberculosis in the United States among foreign-born individuals
in 1987 from selected countries by country of origin.

Country of origin	Percent of all tuberculosis cases in the United States in 1987[8]	Tuberculosis annual case rate per 100,000 in country of origin for 1983-1987[9]
Mexico	5.2	14.7
Philippines	2.8	263.4
Vietnam	1.9	97.9
Haiti	1.4	117.2
Korea	1.3	290.2
India	0.8	114.3

that they can mount against drug-susceptible germs. However, the outcome when disease does develop in normal persons, may not be as benign as that of disease due to drug-susceptible organisms.

A survey was conducted of drug susceptibility and resistance in New York City in April 1991.[10] In that month, five hundred and eighteen patients had cultures from which tubercle bacilli were grown, and studies of drug susceptibility were performed on four hundred and sixty-six of them. One-third of these tuberculosis germs were resistant to the action of one or more of the major drugs used to treat tuberculosis. Nearly one in five were resistant to both isoniazid and rifampin, the two most important tuberculosis treatment drugs. Many of these bacteria came from patients who had been erratic or poorly compliant in their treatment, and it is well known that sporadic pill taking sets the stage for the development of drug resistance of bacteria. So it was that great emphasis came to be placed on assuring that patients completed their initial course of treatment without interruption, using whatever coercive measures might be necessary for noncompliant tuberculosis victims.

Recent information from New York City challenges our thinking about controlling the spread of tuberculosis, and makes even more complex the problem of dealing with multidrug-resistant tuberculosis.

Among persons with newly diagnosed with tuberculosis and taking treatment for the first time, seven percent had MDR organisms.[11] No one can point a finger of shame at these patients and accuse them of failing to cooperate with treatment. They were simply unlucky enough to have been infected with the vicious MDR strain in the first place.

By the early 1990s, many of the MDR tuberculosis cases in New York City, including more than eighty percent of those with organisms resistant to all four of the principal drugs used for treating this disease, were being caused by a germ identified by DNA fingerprinting as one strain, designated strain W. This finding again means that much MDR tuberculosis does not result from failure of patients to follow the dicta of their health care providers. It means that many MDR patients were infected with a bad actor strain of tubercle bacilli from the start and that nothing they or their doctors could do could set aside their misfortune.

Where did strain W come from? Once again, we can develop some clues from the DNA fingerprinting methods borrowed from detectives more commonly seen on the front pages of tabloid newspapers but searching for no less deadly killers. Strain W first appeared in a microepidemic in a hospital in New York in 1990, and it spread rapidly among highly susceptible AIDS patients. However, a close cousin or perhaps the lineal ancestor of this strain has been identified in a patient in Ohio who developed tuberculosis six years earlier. This sleeping beast may have been scattered about the United States, waiting only for a group of AIDS patients to provide the fertile soil for another MDR tuberculosis epidemic. We know that by 1995 patients infected with this strain in New York had subsequently developed tuberculosis in Denver, Atlanta, Miami and Paris.[12] Strain W is on the move.

How did the United States meet the public health challenge presented by its rising epidemic of tuberculosis? Unfortunately, the early response is best described by words such as "poorly" or "belatedly." Just at the time when this national outbreak was mounting, we in America were severely cutting back public health and tuberculosis control program funds. In 1969 more than twenty million federal dollars were allocated to tuberculosis control. By 1982, the figure had fallen to one million dollars.[13]

In 1991, Karen Brudney and Jay Dobkin published a revealing and thought-provoking comparison of the tuberculosis control programs in Sandinista-held Managua, Nicaragua and in New York City.[14] In the wake of war and in the midst of poverty, the Nicaraguans in Managua initiated a program that cured nearly eighty percent of the almost three thousand tuberculosis patients diagnosed annually. At the same time, New York City was able to achieve completion of tuberculosis treatment in only ten to fifteen percent of the cases in poorer neighborhoods—forty percent for the city overall.

How then did the United States face up to its failure to control the ancient scourge of tuberculosis? In the mid and late 1990s, when the problem had become glaringly obvious, our national response shifted, and we attacked the problem with extraordinary if belated vigor, sometimes bordering on panic. Tuberculosis control programs were strengthened and augmented across the nation. Great emphasis was placed on directly observed therapy, being sure that patients complied with their treatment programs. At Goldwater Hospital in New York, a detention ward was opened so that recalcitrant patients could be confined while they completed therapy. Moreover, efforts to reach out to patients under treatment were intensified, and the rate of completion of treatment in New York City climbed to reach ninety percent in 1996.[15] And, in 1993, tuberculosis case rates in America began to decline again. By 1995 the new case rate had fallen to an all time low of 8.7/100,000/year. Perhaps our reinvigorated programs were having an effect. Perhaps the tide was receding.

Only a small portion of the world's tuberculosis occurs in the United States and other technologically advanced countries. Globally, the problem is immense. Tuberculosis is the most important infectious disease in the world. One-third of the people living on Earth are infected with the tubercle bacillus. In 1990, seven and one-half million people developed tuberculosis and two and one-half million people died of this disease.[16] As of that date, tuberculosis caused more deaths in adults than AIDS, leprosy, parasitic diseases, malaria, diarrhea, and acute respiratory infections combined; the surging AIDS epidemic may make it an equally or more important cause of death in the future. More women in the child-bearing age group die of tuberculosis than of complications of pregnancy and child birth.

The major hot spots of the tuberculosis world are in Subsaharan Africa and Southeast Asia. AIDS has resulted in enormous increases in tuberculosis in tropical Africa, and as AIDS spreads to Asia, tuberculosis will follow. In Africa, tuberculosis is the number one infectious complication of AIDS, causing about forty percent of deaths in AIDS patients. Two-thirds of tuberculosis patients in Uganda have AIDS. Haiti also has very high tuberculosis rates, and about one-third of patients there also suffer from AIDS. Even without AIDS, the high mountainous regions of the Andes and the Himalayas have high tuberculosis case rates, and China hosts large numbers of patients with this disease.

The situation is getting worse. In 2005, there will be nearly twelve million new cases of new tuberculosis, and the disease is expected to kill three and one-half million people.[17] These figures represent increases of fifty-eight and thirty-nine percent, respectively. The tide of tuberculosis, which is now ebbing in the United States and Europe, is still to crest in much of the world. In many places, its normal course has been disturbed by the AIDS epidemic, which epidemiologists predict will cause a six-fold increase in tuberculosis in Central Africa during the upcoming decade. In fact, it is the impact of AIDS on tuberculosis, which is discussed more fully in Chapter 17, that has turned world-wide trends of receding tuberculosis incidence into new surges of spreading plague.

What can the future hold? The history of tuberculosis suggests that the current wave will pass, even in the face of AIDS, although many will lie dead in its wake. Our challenge is to lower its crest and hasten its passing.

PART II

The Great White Plague
The Infectious Nature of Tuberculosis

The Microbe is so very small
You cannot make him out at all,
But many sanguine people hope
To see him through a microscope.
His jointed tongue that lies beneath
A hundred curious rows of teeth;
His seven tufted tails with lots
Of lovely pink and purple spots,
On each of which a pattern stands,
Composed of forty separate bands;
His eyebrows of a tender green;
All these have never yet been seen—
But Scientists, who ought to know,
Assure us that they must be so . . .
Oh! let us never, never doubt
What nobody is sure about!

Hilaire Belloc[1]

7

Etude

Frédéric Chopin was born in Zelazowa Wola, Poland on February 22, 1810, the second of four children and the only boy.[2] His mother was a housekeeper for Countess Ludwika Skarbek. His father was a tutor to the countess; he came to Poland to accept that post and there met and married Frédéric's mother. It was a tumultuous and strife-riven time in Poland. Napoleon occupied Warsaw in February 1815, and Czar Alexander of Russia declared himself King of Poland later that same year. While the French and Russians fought, guerrilla bands roamed the country. Chopin's story provides interesting insights into the dawning of the realization that tuberculosis is an infectious disease.

As a boy, the young Chopin was thin, but apparently healthy. At age sixteen, he spent five weeks at a spa in Reinerz, but it is not clear that an illness prompted this interlude. However, tuberculosis was not far away, and in February 1827, when Frédéric was approaching seventeen, his sister, Emilia, developed fulminating tuberculosis. The teen-age boy was greatly affected by her illness, which he described in a letter written March 14, 1827 as follows:

> "We have illness in the house. Emilja has been in bed for four weeks; she has got a cough and has begun to spit blood and Mamma is frightened. Malcz ordered bloodletting. They bled her once, twice; leeches without end, vesicators, sinapisms, wolfsbane; horrors, horrors! — All this time she has been eating nothing; she has grown so thin that you wouldn't know her, and is only now beginning to come to herself a little — You can imagine what it has been like in the house. You'll have to imagine it, because I can't describe it for you."[3]

Did Chopin become infected from his sister? Or perhaps both Frédéric and Emilia became infected from a common source—perhaps from

another household member. Either explanation seems reasonable. However, Chopin would not have believed this hypothesis, for, as we shall
see, tuberculosis was not then thought of as an infectious disease by
Chopin and his northern European contemporaries.

By age nineteen Chopin was recognized as an exceptionally talented
pianist and composer. In 1831, like many Poles of the time, he emigrated to Paris. In Paris, he shared quarters with Jan Matuszynski, a
boyhood friend who had become a physician and was practicing in
Paris. Chopin was rapidly accepted and acclaimed by the musical community of Paris, the arts center of the western world. His first few years
in Paris were probably the happiest ones of his life.

In November 1835 Chopin developed his first overt symptoms of
tuberculosis, with fever, cough, and bloody sputum. His doctor friend,
Jan Matuszynski, prescribed a series of baths, but apparently did not
consider his illness serious. Two years later, he had a relapse, again with
fever, cough, and bloody sputum. He consulted a Dr. Gaubert, who
advised fresh air, exercise, and rest. Dr. Gaubert told him he did not
have tuberculosis and indicated that fresh air would help to prevent
him from contracting the disease. From today's perspective, this advice
seems curious, for we recognize the coughing of blood—hemoptysis, in
medical terms—as a cardinal sign of pulmonary tuberculosis. But many
doctors of Chopin's time did not make this association, and hemoptysis
was thought to be a possible cause of consumption, rather than a symptom of it.

In 1836, Franz Liszt, Chopin's compatriot and great friend, introduced him to George Sand. She was a leading literary figure in her
time, who to this day ranks as a superb writer. She was taken with him
immediately, calling him "a poor melancholy angel." Thin and chronically ill, he fit well into the glamorized, romanticized image of a consumptive. Chopin appears to have had little romantic interest in Sand
initially, but their relationship blossomed, and by the autumn of 1838
they were lovers.

Concerned for Chopin's health, Sand induced him to travel with her
to Mallorca, a Spanish Mediterranean Island where the couple hoped
that the mild climate would restore Chopin's health and permit him to
pursue his composing with renewed vigor. Chopin was delighted with
what he found on Mallorca. On November 19, 1838, he wrote to Julian

Fontana, his agent in Paris, describing his pleasure with his surroundings.

> "I am in Palma, among palms, cedars, cacti, olives, pomegranates, etc. Everything the *Jardin de Plantes* has in its greenhouses. A sky like turquoise, a sea like lapis lazuli, mountains like emerald, air like heaven. Sun all day, and hot; everyone in summer clothing; at night guitars and singing for hours. Huge balconies with grape-vines overhead; Moorish walls. Everything looks towards Africa, as the town does. In short, a glorious life!"

However, his new-found contentment was short lived. Two weeks later he again wrote to Fontana:

> "I can't send you the manuscript, for it's not finished. I have been as sick as a dog these last two weeks; I caught cold in spite of eighteen degrees of heat, roses, oranges, palms, figs and three most famous doctors of the island. One sniffed at what I spat up, the second tapped where I spat it from, the third poked about and listened how I spat it. One said I had died, the second that I am dying, the 3rd that I shall die. And today I'm the same as ever; only I can't forgive Jasio for not giving me a consultation when I had an attack of *bronchite aigue*, which can always be expected in my case. I could scarcely keep them from bleeding me, and they put no setons or vesicators; but grace to Providence, I am now as before. But all this has affected the Preludes, and God knows when you will get them."

Chopin's reluctance to accept bleeding and blistering from his physicians may have resulted from his memories of his sister's illness and demise and the treatment she received.

The physicians who attended Chopin did more than sniff, tap, and listen. They told the townspeople of Palma that he was a contagious danger in their midst. George Sand, in an eloquent and poignant letter written the following March, after the couple had left Mallorca, described this event as follows:

> " . . . we had succeeded in settling down at Mallorca, a magnificent place, but inhospitable to the utmost degree. At the end of a month, poor Chopin, who had always been coughing from the time we left

Paris, fell more seriously ill, so that we had to call in one, two, three doctors, each more asinine than the others, who went about the island saying that the patient was in the last stage of consumption. This caused great consternation, phthisis being extremely rare in those latitudes, and, moreover, considered contagious! Added to this were the egotism, the cowardice, the want of feeling, and the bad faith of the inhabitants. We were looked upon as pestiferous, and, worse, as heathens, for we did not attend mass. The landlord of the little cottage that we had hired ejected us brutally, and wanted to bring an action against us in order to compel us to whitewash his house, which he pretended was infected. Had he succeeded, the native jurisprudence would have completely skinned us!"[4]

Forced to leave Palma, Chopin and Sand found refuge in Valdemosa, a village overlooking the west coast of the island located at an altitude of about fourteen hundred feet above the sea. George Sand described their exodus to this mountain retreat as follows:

"We had to submit to expulsion, contumely and extortion. Not knowing what to do, for Chopin's state of health did not allow of his being taken back to France, we were delighted to meet, in an old Carthusian convent, a Spanish family whom political reasons had compelled to seek a hiding-place there, and who possessed a tolerably decent suite of peasant furniture. The refugees intended to pass over to France; we, therefore, bought the furniture for three times its value, and installed ourselves in the convent of Valdemosa: a poetical name, a poetical abode—charming scenery, grand and wild, with the sea bordering on the horizon, formidable heights around us, eagles pursuing their prey even into the orange groves of our garden. . . . Nothing could be more magnificent."

Chopin looked forward to the move, writing again to Fontana in Paris on December 14

"Meanwhile my manuscripts sleep, and I can't sleep; only cough and, covered with poultices for a long time past, wait for the spring or for something else—Tomorrow I go to that wonderful monastery of Valdemosa, to write in the cell of some old monk, who perhaps had more fire in his soul than I, and stifled it, stifled and extinguished it, because he had it in vain."

The mountain aerie was less than idyllic. Partly because they did not attend mass and partly because Chopin's disease was feared, the couple was not accepted readily. With great eloquence, George Sand wrote:

"But he was right who laid it down as a principle that whenever nature is gorgeous and beautiful, men are wicked and sordid. There we had all the trouble in the world to procure the commonest necessaries of life, though the island produces them in profusion; . . . We were unable to procure servants, because we were not *Christians*;[5] and besides, nobody cared to wait upon a consumptive person. We, nevertheless, were pretty comfortably lodged. . . ."

Chopin grew worse. The winter weather in the mountains was cloudy and rainy, and the couple believed that the weather and altitude were contributing to his illness. They were discouraged by what they perceived as prejudiced rejection by the people whom they met on Mallorca. And so they decided to leave. Departure, however, was not easy. Again, as described by George Sand:

" . . . .Chopin grew worse daily, and in spite of all the offers of services which the people made us in the *Spanish fashion*, we could not have found a hospitable house in the whole island. We at last decided to go away, at whatever cost, although Chopin had not even strength enough to drag himself along. We requested a simple, a first and last service—a conveyance to Palma, where we intended to embark. That service was refused, although our *friends* all had carriages and a suitable fortune. We were obliged to travel three leagues along outlandish paths in a *birlocho*, that is to say, a wheelbarrow![6]

"Upon reaching Palma, Chopin had a dreadful fit of blood-spitting; the next day we embarked on board the only steamboat in the island, and which is used for the transport of pigs to Barcelona. That was our only means of leaving the accursed country. We travelled in the company of *a hundred pigs*, whose ceaseless grunting and unbearable stench left neither rest nor respirable air for our patient. Chopin arrived at Barcelona still spitting blood by basinsfull, and crawling along like a spectre. There, happily, our misfortunes began to diminish! The French Consul and the Commander of the French Naval Station received us with an hospitality and a graciousness quite unknown in Spain. We were taken on board a beautiful brig belonging to the fleet. The surgeon, a brave and worthy man, at once came to the assistance of the patient, and in twenty-four hours stopped the hemorrhage of the lung."

Chopin and Sand embarked by sea for Marseilles. During the trip, Chopin had another major pulmonary hemorrhage. But after arrival in Marseilles, his bleeding stopped and he began to improve. In the words of George Sand:

"Chopin bore the sea passage very well. He is now, very weak, though infinitely better in all respects, and in the hands of Dr. Cauvière, an excellent doctor, who tends him like a father, and pledges himself for his recovery. We are at length breathing freely, but after what trouble and anguish!"

That spring, Chopin wrote to Fontana:

"I am much better. I am beginning to play, eat, walk, and talk, like other folk; you see that I even write easily, since you again receive a few words from me."

In May, Chopin and Sand went to her family home in Nohant, where they spent the next several summers. Winters were passed in Paris. Chopin became part of the Sand family, and developed a close relationship with Sand's daughter, Solange Clésinger. Ultimately, it was Chopin's defense of Solange in a dispute with her mother that precipitated the end of the lovers' deteriorating relationship in 1846.

Meanwhile, Chopin continued to compose and perform, although frequently ill. The winter of 1844 was particularly difficult for him; he signed two love letters written that December to Sand:

"Always yours, older than ever; very, extremely, incredibly old. . . . Ch."

and

"Your mummified ancient, Ch."

After a bitter parting from George Sand in 1846, Chopin stayed on in Paris. In a Christmas letter written to his family in Poland in 1847, Chopin seemed resigned to his ill health, rather than concerned about it:

"Meanwhile, the winter here is not very good. There is a great deal of grippe, but I have enough with my usual cough, and am no more afraid of grippe than you of cholera. I smell my homeopathic flasks from time to time, give many lessons in the house, and manage as I can."

However, the seesaw course of his battle with tuberculosis continued. In February of 1848 he gave a concert in Paris, his first in six years and the last he was to give in Paris. While the concert was received with enthusiasm, Chopin was hardly able to enjoy his success. He collapsed at the end of the performance and had to be helped from the stage. He canceled a performance scheduled for the following month.

In April, Chopin went to London. He gave several successful concerts, one of which was attended by Queen Victoria and Prince Albert. That summer he moved to Edinburgh, Scotland, staying with a Mrs. Stirling, a former pupil who was enamored of him and hoped to marry him. Chopin did not return her affections. Neither the Scottish weather nor social life agreed with Chopin, and on August 19 he wrote to a Polish friend:

" . . . I am fit for nothing now; and then, when I dress, everything strains me, and I gasp that way till dinner time. Afterwards one has to sit two hours at table with the men, look at them talking and listen to them drinking. I am bored to death (I am thinking of one thing and they of another, in spite of all their courtesy and French remarks at table). Then I go to the drawing-room, where it takes all my efforts to be a little animated—because they usually want to hear me—; then my good Daniel carries me up to my bedroom (as you know that is usually upstairs here), undresses me, gets me to bed, leaves the light; and I am free to breathe and dream till it is time to begin all over again."

Chopin's illness progressed, and he became confined to bed. He consulted Sir James Clark, the royal court physician, and a leading authority on tuberculosis.[7] Clark did not believe in the infectious nature of tuberculosis and considered the prevailing Southern European view "obsolete." Clark based his treatment of consumption on travel to mild climates. In Chopin's words, Clark "gave him his benediction."

On November 16, 1848, Chopin roused himself to give his last public performance at a benefit ball for Polish exiles. Soon thereafter, discouraged, he decided to return to a Paris apartment in the Place d'Orléans. In a letter to Sand's daughter, Solange, he wrote:

> "Tomorrow I go to Paris, scarcely dragging myself, and weaker than you have ever seen me. The doctors are driving me away from here. I am swollen up with neuralgia, can neither breathe nor sleep, and have not left my room since November 1st (except the 16th, to play for an hour in the evening at the concert for the Poles). After that I relapsed; I cannot possibly breathe here . . ."

In Paris, he remained bedridden, unable to compose or write, destitute and dependent upon the generosity of his friends. He was not only wasting from tuberculosis, but he was in respiratory and cardiac failure, the consequences of the advanced state of his disease. In June 1849 he suffered a devastating series of pulmonary hemorrhages, and on June 25 he wrote to his family in Poland asking them to come to him. By the fall he was obviously dying. His last written words, scribbled to a friend with a pencil on a piece of note paper when he was too weak to speak were:

> "As this cough will choke me, I implore you to have my body opened, so that I may not be buried alive."

On October 15, 1849 Chopin asked for a priest, who administered the last rites of the Church. His physician, a Dr. Cruveilhier,[8] attended him on his death bed. On October 17, 1849 after a long fit of coughing, Dr. Cruveilhier asked Chopin if he suffered. Faintly, Frédéric Chopin replied "plus"—no more, his last words.

8

Animalcula

George Sand was indignant that Frédéric Chopin's tuberculosis was considered contagious by the residents of Mallorca. Sir James Clark, physician to both Chopin and Keats, considered the belief that tuberculosis was infectious to be obsolete. What led these people to be so badly mistaken about one of the most ancient and widespread infections of humans? In fact, their viewpoints were not unusual in their time, and it is worth considering how the notion that tuberculosis or any disease could be transmitted from person to person came to be accepted and then established as fact.

As we have seen, Hippocrates knew tuberculosis well. He noted the small tuberculomas ($\phi\hat{v}\mu\alpha\tau\alpha$) in diseased lungs that are typical manifestations of tuberculosis, and he considered them to be the cause rather than the result of this disease. He did not consider tuberculosis infectious. Indeed, the entire concept of infectious diseases was lacking at that time. One of Hippocrates's contemporaries, the historian Thucydides, did embrace the notion that disease could be transmitted from person to person in his description of a plague that swept through Athens. The nature of this epidemic is not known; it could have been any one of many contagious diseases. Five centuries later, the great Greco-Roman physician Galen appears to have clearly understood that tuberculosis was transmitted from person to person.

Few new ideas developed during the middle ages, but in the middle of the thirteenth century Pietro Curialti de Tossignano emphasized the spread of tuberculosis by contact in his writings. In the following century, plague—"the black death"—swept across Europe, and contact with diseased or deceased persons was widely thought to be important in becoming ill. In 1546, Hieronymus Frascatorius of Verona, who lived from 1484 to 1553, wrote a work entitled "The Theory of Infection," in which he clearly recognized that infections could be passed from one individual to another.[1] He also attributed the spread of contagious diseases to fomites, which he described as "clothing, screens and other things healthy in themselves but apt to conserve the first seeds of infection and to infect through them."[2] Frascatorius came to recognize that some diseases might be spread by the aerial route, but he did not consider this route of infection important. He did not include tuberculosis among the infectious diseases he catalogued.[3]

Daniel Defoe, the author of *Robinson Crusoe*, was born in 1661. When he was four years old, an epidemic of plague swept London. Years later, in 1722, Defoe published a vivid account of that epidemic. In it he refers to the killing of "forty thousand dogs, and five times as many cats. . . . All possible endeavours were us'd also to destroy mice and rats, especially the latter, . . . and a prodigious multitude of them were also destroy'd."[4] Plague, of course, was spread by fleas living on rats.

Writing in 1680, Franciscus Sylvius, of French birth but living in Germany, described the characteristic tubercles in the lungs of patients with tuberculosis. "It is known this disease can be hereditary," he stated, "transmitted from parents to children; but in whatever this hereditary consists, is also not known." About the same time, Richard Morton, a leading English medical practitioner who later became physician to the king, described several causes of tuberculosis, including "a foggy and thick air, and that which is filled with the smoak of coals, . . . an hereditary disposition from the parents, . . . and an ill formation of the breast."[5] Thus, during the seventeenth century, when the tuberculosis epidemic was escalating rapidly in northern Europe, tuberculosis and most other infectious diseases were not generally thought to be contagious. The prevailing view was that tuberculosis was hereditary. For only a few other diseases, such as syphilis and plague, had the concept of contagion emerged.

In 1720, a remarkable book was published in London. It was written by Benjamin Marten, the son of a poor tailor who acquired a knowledge of apothecary lore early in his life and who earned a medical degree from the University of Edinburgh in 1717. Little is known about his life, but it is apparent that he was familiar with the earlier microscopy work of van Leeuwenhoek, who is often credited with the discovery of the microscope and who described microorganisms, designating them "animalcula." In his book, entitled "A New Theory of Consumptions: More Especially of a Phthisis or Consumption of the Lungs," Marten first provided a lucid description of pulmonary tuberculosis and then posited that tuberculosis was caused by animalcula:

> "The *Original* and *Essential Cause*, then, which some content themselves to call a vicious Disposition of the Juices, others a salt Acrimony, others a strange Ferment, others a malignant Humor (all of which seem to me dark and unintelligible) may possibly be some certain species of *Animalcula* or wonderfully minute living Creatures, that, by their peculiar Shape, or disagreeable Parts, are inimicable to our Nature; but however capable of subsisting in our Juices and Vessels, and which being drove to the Lungs by the Circulation of the Blood, . . . may be then . . . stimulating, and perhaps wounding or gnawing the tender Vessels of the Lungs, caus(ing) all the Disorders that have been mentioned. . . ."

Clearly Marten embraced a germ theory of disease not far from modern concepts and applied this theory to tuberculosis.[6]

René T. H. Laennec was a French physician who lived from 1781 to 1826. His published autopsy studies of tuberculosis are lucid and even today stand as examples of clear medical writing.[7] Most importantly, it was Laennec's work that firmly established that tuberculosis appearing in many forms and in many parts of the body did, indeed, represent a single disease. However, some did not accept Laennec's conclusions, most notably Virchow, the most famous and respected pathologist of the nineteenth century.

Laennec rejected many of the contemporary views of the cause of tuberculosis, but concluded that the cause was unknowable. Interestingly, his own experience proved the infectious nature of this disease, although he did not recognize it. At age twenty-five, he cut his hand while doing an autopsy on a person who had died of tuberculosis. He then developed a chronic tuberculous lesion at the site of the cut—a "prosector's wart." The lesion ultimately healed and remained healed.[8] Despite Laennec's ability to control the local tuberculous infection of his hand, his body did not control the disease elsewhere; Laennec died of tuberculosis at age forty-five.

It was Jean-Antoine Villemin, a French military surgeon, who finally established convincingly that tuberculosis is infectious and that it is one disease wherever it occurs in the body. He inoculated rabbits with material from tuberculous lesions of humans and induced similar lesions in the rabbits. He described his experiments as follows:

"March 6, 1865, we took two rabbits about three weeks old, very heathy, . . . In one of these rabbits, we introduced into a little subcutaneous wound behind each ear, two small fragments of tubercle and a small amount of purulent liquid from a tuberculous cavity, removed from the lung and the intestine of a consumptive, who had been dead twenty-three hours.

"June 20th, that is, at the end of three months and fourteen days, there was no appreciable change in the health of the animal, . . . (and so) we sacrificed it and noted the following:

"The lungs are full of large tubercular masses, formed, in an obvious manner, from the agglomeration of numerous granulations; . . . The other rabbit, who had shared the same conditions of life with the inoculated rabbit, . . . did not show a single tubercle."[9]

Villemin's description of his work is elegant; it would stand critical review by modern standards. The stage was set for Koch's discovery of the tubercle bacillus to come seventeen years later. However, the eminent German pathologist Virchow remained unconvinced.

Why did Villemin's inoculated rabbit remain healthy after it developed tuberculosis? That is a story that harkens forward to the work of Lurie, which is discussed in Chapter 14. Rabbits are singularly resistant to human tuberculosis. Had Villemin chosen to inoculate guinea pigs or monkeys, the outcome probably would have been very different.

Meanwhile, the concept that tuberculosis was, indeed, infectious and that persons ill with tuberculosis constituted a public health threat had become well established in southern Europe. In 1699, the Republic of Lucca in Italy issued an edict requiring that "the health of the human body shall not be harmed or imperiled by . . . a person infected with the disease of phthisis, and physicians must give notice of persons . . . they shall have treated for the suspected malady." Ventilation of the rooms of patients with tuberculosis was required as well as cleaning of the patients effects and living quarters. Spain required notification of all contagious cases of tuberculosis in 1751. Physicians who failed to report their patients were fined or imprisoned. In the 1780s, laws were passed in Italy that required reporting of tuberculous patients by physicians, with fines or banishment specified for physicians who failed to comply; cleaning or burning of the clothing and personal effects of persons who died of tuberculosis; and replastering of houses occupied by tuberculous patients, with the house then to remain vacant for six months.[10]

George Sand thought the people of Mallorca to be inhospitable. Perhaps they were, but they were doing no more than they believed to be proper for the protection of the health of the public. The early Italian and Spanish laws presaged public health measures later employed in Europe and North America—but not until after the passing of a century and a half. The first regulations requiring reporting of tuberculosis in England were enacted in 1903.[11] Similar rules were promulgated in other northern European countries about the same time.

Norman Bethune was an idealistic communist North American thoracic surgeon who fought with the loyalists in the Spanish revolution of 1936 and led the medical services suporting Mao's Eighth Route Army in China. He is to this day a hero in China. His flamboyant career was interrupted by tuberculosis in 1927, and he spent a year at the Trudeau Sanatorium in Saranac Lake. Living in one of Trudeau's cottages, he papered his walls with murals drawn on the paper that wrapped his laundry. In these murals, he depicted tubercle bacilli as long tailed red bats—fanciful animalcula.[12]

Robert Koch and the Tubercle Bacillus

Robert Koch was an extraordinary person and certainly the most important figure in the history of tuberculosis. His contributions to our knowledge of tuberculosis and the science of microbiology were enormous and without equal, before or since. In fact, one might well argue that he was one of the greatest contributors to medical knowledge of all time. Single handedly, he discovered the cause of tuberculosis. Who was this genius?

Heinrich Herrmann Robert Koch was born in Clausthal, Lower Saxony, on December 11, 1843. He was the third of thirteen children, eleven of whom survived to adulthood. His father was a mining engineer. His mother favored her third son, Robert, but in this busy household, it was his mother's brother, Eduard Biewend, who befriended the boy and stimulated his interest both in nature and photography. The young Koch collected insects and plants, and his daily chores included care of the family's barnyard animals.[1] He was precocious, learning to read at age five. Despite his obvious intelligence, he was a desultory student, and he earned only average grades at school. He played chess. He enjoyed music, and he played both the piano and the zither.

Koch's two older brothers emigrated to the United States. His father offered him the chance to join them. Koch declined, however, perhaps because of his growing infatuation with Emmy Fraatz, whom he later married. Instead, at age nineteen, Koch entered the university at Gottingen.

Gottingen had a distinguished faculty, and the studies Koch undertook there had a profound influence on his later life. Koch later reflected that his greatest teachers were Jacob Henle, a distinguished pathologist who had come to accept the germ theory of infectious diseases; Karl Hasse, a clinician; and Georg Meissner, a physiologist and animal experimentalist. Others clearly also influenced him. With Meissner and also with Wilhelm Krause, a pathologist, Koch carried out experimental studies while a student. He won a student research prize, and he published two scientific papers while still a university student. In 1886 at age twenty-three, he received his doctorate in medicine *maxima cum laude*. His thesis concerned succinic acid metabolism, and he served as his own experimental subject for many of his studies.

Upon leaving the university, Koch passed his medical licensure examination and assumed a staff position at the Hamburg General Hospital. His childhood sweetheart, Emmy Fraatz, accepted his proposal of marriage. Koch found himself in need of more money, and in October he left Hamburg to take a better paying position in nearby Langenhagen at an institution for retarded children. Koch opened a private medical practice in Langenhagen as well, and he soon found himself busy with a thriving practice. On July 16, 1867, he and Emmy were married in the church in Clausthal. There was no honeymoon, however, for Koch had to return to Langenhagen shortly after the ceremony to attend a sick patient.

The next two years were happy ones for Robert and Emmy. However, budget cut-backs led to the end of his employment at the Langenhagen institution, and Koch found himself hard pressed to meet his financial obligations. Emmy was pregnant; she gave birth to their daughter Gertrude on September 6, 1868. Koch left Langenhagen, and tried to establish practices in other small communities, but without success. He was in financial straits, and his relationship with Emmy had begun to deteriorate. Finally, in July 1869, he opened a successful practice in Rakwitz, Posen (now a part of Poland).

War broke out with France, and in 1870 Robert Koch and three of his younger brothers volunteered for military service. Koch was rejected because of his poor eyesight. The following year, Koch volunteered again, and this time was accepted for limited duty. He was assigned to a battlefield hospital, and as the German army rolled across eastern France, Koch went with it, serving with his hospital unit in Neufchatel and Orleans. However, even before the war ended, Koch returned to resume his practice in Rakwitz, as there was a pressing need for a doctor there. Koch's army experience had a great effect on him. He became profoundly nationalistic and violently anti-French. This feeling persisted into his later years, and it led him to spurn Louis Pasteur, his great French contemporary.

Koch had had a continuing interest in a position as a district medical officer, and he had taken and passed the qualifying examination for such a post. In April 1872 he accepted this position at Wollstein, a town of about four thousand people in the Polish part of Prussia. The position provided a salary and also permitted him to have a private practice. Koch's duties included serving as public health officer for Wollstein, giving small pox vaccinations, writing death certificates, and overseeing the local hospital. His practice was successful, and he became a revered physician in the community. A patient later wrote of him, "What a doctor! There was something special about him. How often did I hear my mother say: 'If Dr. Koch came into your sick room, you immediately felt calm and secure.'"[2]

Koch's house at Wollstein was commodious, and it included a large back room that served as the consultation room for his practice. He soon partitioned it with a curtain, half for his clinic, half for his laboratory. It was in this laboratory that most of Koch's pioneering work was carried out. He equipped it with an incubator, a sink, and a work bench. After careful budgeting by the two of them, his wife Emmy gave him a microscope. This extravagant purchase, so important to his pioneering bacteriological studies, was chosen over a carriage, which would have provided comfortable transportation for both husband and wife and greatly facilitated the house calls Koch made on sick patients in the rural area surrounding Wollstein.

Robert Koch's life at Wollstein was not only productive; it was also happy. Koch made friends in the community, and joined them in local taverns. He and Emmy shared an amateur interest in archeology, and they assisted in excavations at a local archeologic site. The married couple clearly had some difficulties, but Emmy assisted Robert in his experiments, and they purchased Koch's microscope together as a twenty-eighth birthday gift from her to him. Koch built a dark room and pursued his hobby of photography. His daughter, who now bore the nickname Trudy, was growing up, and Koch was enchanted with her.

Koch's early laboratory studies focused on the techniques of bacteriology. Pasteur had demonstrated that bacteria could produce fermentation and were responsible for turning wine to vinegar. Pasteur also identified bacteria causing a disease in silk worms that had become a major problem for silk producers in France. Koch knew of Pasteur's work, and he remained under the influence of Jacob Henle, his university professor. Thus, Koch did not work in an intellectual void. However, existing techniques were crude and inadequate for many important studies. Koch invented a number of procedures that still underlie modern microbiological techniques.

Koch turned his attention to anthrax, an important disease of sheep and cattle and sometimes of humans. Other scientists of the time had observed bacteria in the blood of some diseased animals with anthrax, but they were puzzled by the absence of these bacteria in other ill animals. Koch cultured the anthrax bacillus[3] in drops of liquid medium hanging from thin glass microscope cover slips, an imaginative technique that permitted him to observe the life cycle of the bacterium through his microscope. He observed that the anthrax bacillus developed spores, and then found these spores in the blood of those animals in which the entire bacillus had not been seen by his colleagues. These studies convincingly established the bacteriologic cause of anthrax, perhaps the first firm demonstration of the cause of any infectious disease.

Koch photographed his hanging drop cultures through his microscope, the first use of photomicrography. In April of 1876 Koch presented his findings, including the photographs, to the faculty of the Institute of Plant Science in Breslau. The importance of his work was recognized immediately. One of the scientists there is said to have summoned his laboratory staff, "drop everything and go listen to Koch. . . . There is nothing left to prove. I regard it as the greatest discovery ever made with microorganisms."[4] The director of the institute, Ferdinand Cohn, published Koch's paper in the next issue of the scientific journal he edited.

One individual remained unconvinced by Koch's experiments. Rudolf Virchow, the leading pathologist of the time, one of Europe's best-known scientists, and to this day a revered person in the annals of pathology, did not accept the germ theory of disease. Koch presented his results to the sceptical Virchow who rebuffed him, and from this time forward the two men had an increasingly distant and sometimes antagonistic relationship.

Cohn offered Koch a post at the Breslau institute, but Koch stayed there only three months before returning to Wollstein. Cohn then proposed Koch for an appointment at the Imperial Health Office in Berlin, where a laboratory and research funds were provided for him in 1880. Koch's innovations and contributions to the emerging science of bacteriology during the next few years were remarkable. In studying anthrax he had developed the hanging drop culture technique and taken the first photomicrographs of bacteria. He went on to invent the method of steam sterilization. He worked in partnership with Ernst Abbe at Carl Zeiss, the famous lens makers, and he was the first to use oil immersion lenses and the new substage optical condenser developed by Abbe. Koch showed that staphylococci and streptococci ("staph" and "strep" are so well known today they are household words; they were newly discovered at that time) were causes of wound infections. He developed solid culture media that for the first time allowed the culture of pure strains of bacteria. In August of 1881 he attended the International Medical Congress in London and presented his work. There are no formal records of that meeting, but it was apparently Koch's demonstation of his solid culture media for bacterial growth that excited the assembled scientists. At the end of his lecture, Louis Pasteur, his French rival and some twenty years his senior, went to the front of the hall, took Koch's hand, and congratulated him, "C'est un grand progrès!"—this is a great advance![5] There were greater advances to come.

In August 1881, shortly after his return from London, Koch began work in his new Berlin laboratory on tuberculosis. He was aided by laboratory assistants, whom his modest research budget allowed him to hire. His first two assistants were Friedrich Loeffler and Georg Gaffky, both of whom went on to be famous in their own right, Loeffler principally for discovering the cause of diphtheria and Gaffky for identifying the cause of typhoid. Today, the name of Gaffky is still known to microbiologists, for it is attached to a standard scale for describing the number of tubercle bacilli present in sputum from patients with tuberculosis.

The pace of work by Koch and his assistants was extraordinary, considering the relatively long time it takes to grow tubercle bacilli.[6] The speed of his investigations is even more remarkable when one realizes that Koch and his assistants used many innovative techniques that he had only recently developed or that they developed during the course of this work. Koch appears to have worked largely in secrecy, not inform-

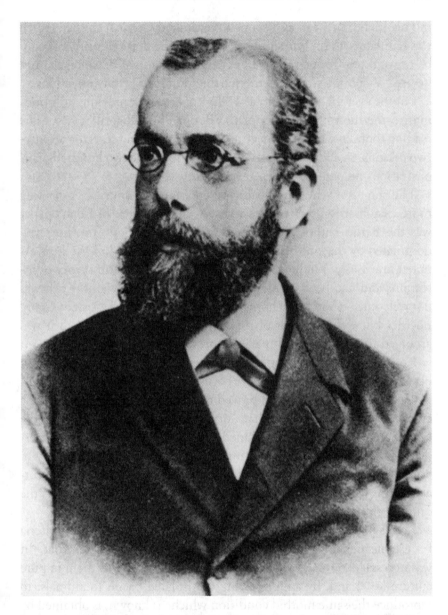

Figure 9.1. Robert Koch. this photograph was taken in 1883, the year following his report of his discovery of the tubercle bacillus.

ing his friend, mentor, and sponsor Ferdinand Cohn at Breslau. Koch was familiar with the work of Villemin showing that tuberculosis could be transmitted from an infected person to an animal (Chapter 8), and he used Villemin's studies as the starting point for his investigations.

On the evening of March 24, 1882 Robert Koch presented his findings to the monthly meeting of the Berlin Physiological Society. The reading room in which the meeting was convened had seats for seventy-two persons. In addition, tables were set up for some two hundred demonstrations prepared by Koch. Every seat was taken.[7]

The choice of venue for Koch's presentation was unusual. A meeting more customarily used for presentations of the nature of Koch's paper was the Berlin Pathological Society. The latter society was, however, dominated by the eminent Professor of Pathology, Rudolf Virchow. As noted previously, Virchow had not yet accepted the germ theory of infections and had been highly critical of Koch's earlier work. Koch was not welcome on Virchow's home turf. Koch's friend and assistant Georg Loeffler knew the director of the Physiological Society, and so it was arranged that Koch would make his presentation there.

Koch made his presentation in a quiet voice; he was not and never became a facile public speaker. He began by acknowledging the work of Villemin and others who had proved the transmissible nature of tuberculosis. He went on to note that, "one-seventh of all human beings die of tuberculosis." As Koch continued, it was soon apparent that his message was an extraordinary one. In this paper, entitled "The Etiology of Tuberculosis,"[8] Koch demonstrated with great clarity and in unrefutable terms that the tubercle bacillus, *Mycobacterium tuberculosis*,[9] is the cause of tuberculosis.

Koch's paper made three major points. First he described his criteria for establishing that a bacterium caused a disease. He stated that, "it was necessary to isolate the bacilli from the body; to grow them in pure culture . . . ; and, by administering the isolated bacilli to animals, to reproduce the same morbid condition which, as known, is obtained by inoculation with spontaneously developed tuberculous material."[10] Modified and elaborated upon only slightly in subsequent decades, these criteria have come to be known as Koch's postulates and are still in use by scientists today. It has been pointed out that these postulates were extensions of those previously posed by Jacob Henle, one of Koch's university professors at Gottingen. While this is true, Koch's statement had remarkable clarity—more than the earlier writings of Henle—and history has chosen to attach Koch's name rather than that of Henle to these famous postulates.

Secondly, Koch described tubercle bacilli and the means by which he stained and cultured them. He described his extensive animal experiments, in which his postulates were fulfilled. Finally, Koch described the reactions of animals inoculated with tubercle bacilli. His experiments in this latter area were pioneering and set the stage for the development of new knowledge about resistance to tuberculosis. This aspect of tuberculosis is discussed in Part III of this book.

The reaction to Koch's presentation was one of awe. In place of the customary polite applause, there was silence born of amazement. One attendee later wrote, "the audience was left spellbound, and for a time after he had ended the presentation not a word was uttered."[11] There is an apocryphal story that Rudolf Virchow was in the audience and that it was customary for that contemporary master of the science pathology to ask the first question at such presentations. Virchow sat silent, so the story goes, stunned by the unassailability of Koch's work and knowing that he must now accept both the tenet that tuberculosis in all organs is a single disease and that Koch's bacillus is its cause. It is more likely, however, that Virchow was not present at Koch's presentation. Carter, a major biographer and translator of Koch, quotes directly from an observer that, "Virchow was conspicuously absent."[12]

Word of Koch's discoveries spread rapidly. The paper he presented was published on April 10, 1882 in *Berliner Klinische Wochenschrift*. The discovery was announced in *The Times* of London in a letter from Koch's English colleague John Tyndall on April 23, and Tyndall's letter was reprinted by the *New York Times* on May 3. An editorial in the *New York Times* on May 7 complained of the delay in transmitting the important news to North America.[13] Paul Ehrlich, a distinguished chemist who heard Koch's presentation, repeated his stains and then improved upon them. Edward Livingston Trudeau, who had recently opened his laboratory in Saranac Lake, New York, repeated and confirmed some of Koch's experiments. He described Koch's paper as "certainly one of the most, if not the most, important medical papers ever written."[14] Seldom before or since has a scientific discovery been so rapidly accepted.

Seldom since has a discovery of such importance to the health of the world been announced.

Koch was instantly famous and widely heralded as the preeminent German scientist of the day. Honors came his way, one after another. Ultimately, Germany would build a new research Institute for Infectious Diseases in Berlin for Koch.

Cholera—the dread epidemic diarrheal disease that had spread in deadly waves across the world repeatedly through history—had resurfaced in Egypt and India, and cases had started to appear in Europe. Confident that the new science of microbiology could deal with all disease problems, European nations organized research teams to investigate the cause of cholera. Koch was asked to assume command of the German team, and he quickly assembled a team of German scientists and a mobile laboratory and left for Egypt. A French team, headed by Koch's rival Pasteur, reached Egypt two weeks before the Germans. Both scientific teams began by using microscopes to look for a germ in specimens from cholera patients and both tried to culture a germ. Both the Germans and French described bacteria, but it was obvious they were looking at different organisms. Koch described the organism his team saw as like a comma. Neither team was able to culture the organisms they saw.

The cholera epidemic waned in Egypt, and the European scientists were unable to obtain fresh specimens for study. Pasteur and his colleagues returned to Paris. Koch and the other Germans, however, moved on to India to continue their investigations. In Bombay, Koch again identified his comma-like bacterium in all fresh cases of cholera, and he now succeeded in growing it in cultures. *Vibrio cholera*[15] had been found, and Koch was certain it was the cause of cholera. Although history proved Koch correct, he was disappointed that he could not reproduce the disease in experimental animals. Cholera germs simply do not cause disease in most animals. Koch returned to Berlin triumphantly. It seemed he could do no wrong, could solve any problem.

Koch continued his studies of tuberculosis, and his famous postulates, first presented in his dramatic paper in 1882, were further refined. Ultimately, they were stated in the form best known today not by Koch but by his associate Georg Loeffler in his description of the cause of diphtheria:[16]

1. The organism must be shown to be constantly present in . . . diseased tissue.
2. The organism . . . must be isolated and grown in pure culture.
3. The (organism grown in) pure culture must be shown to induce the disease experimentally.

Late in 1889, Koch abandoned his administrative desk and public life to return to his laboratory. He worked alone and in secrecy. The first clue to his activities emerged on August 3, 1890. Koch delivered an invited lecture to the Tenth International Congress of Medicine, which was held in Berlin. He stated that he had "found substances that halted the growth of tuberculosis bacilli not only in test tubes but also in animal bodies."[17] He did not elaborate in much detail, and he made no further public statements on the matter until November 15, 1890. On that date he published a three page paper in *Deutsche Medicinische Wochenschrift*.[18] In this paper, Koch drew two major conclusions. First he observed that previously infected animals and persons with tuberculosis reacted more vigorously to the substance he injected than did uninfected individuals. Thus, his substance might have "diagnostic value;" this aspect of Koch's observations is discussed in Chapter 13. Secondly, Koch concluded that his material protected animals from tuberculosis and promoted the healing of tuberculous lesions; the story of this "curative effect" is treated in Chapter 20. Koch did not reveal the nature of his material, except that it was "a suspension of glycerin and extracts from tubercle bacilli cultures."

The response to Koch's announcement was extraordinary. Both patients and doctors flocked to Berlin. Koch distributed his fluid widely. Clinical trials were undertaken, but these were not well designed and the results are difficult to interpret today. The material came to be called tuberculin, and the medical world was split on whether it was proper or not for Koch to keep its nature secret. An editorial in the Journal of the American Medical Association concluded that Koch's secrecy was probably the result of orders from his superiors in the German government, who wished to be sure that unscrupulous imitators did not produce "spurious Koch's fluid."[19] Finally, in October 1891, Koch published a paper in which he reported more extensively on his studies, described the results of treating tuberculous patients with his fluid, and revealed that his tuberculin was nothing more than the concentrated glycerin-rich medium of liquid cultures that had been heat-killed and filtered.[20]

Within a year it became apparent that Koch's tuberculin was not the curative agent he had hoped for. Koch struggled with more and more experiments, adding to knowledge about immunity to tuberculosis, but coming no closer to his therapeutic goal. One of his major collaborators, Emil von Behring, left Koch's laboratory to pursue his own career, and became a rival; bitter relationships between the former colleagues developed. Koch's beloved daughter Trudy had married Eduard Pfuhl, one of Koch's research assistants in 1888, and Koch was "not completely overjoyed" by the marriage.[21] Koch's long strained relationship with his wife, Emmy deteriorated further.

In 1890 or 1891, Koch met a young art student named Hedwig Freiberg. She was seventeen, and captivated by the famous scientist. Within months, they were lovers. The scientific community was scandalized. The famous pathologist Metchnikoff noted, "During the Congress of German Physicians in 1892, . . . Koch's marriage was the topic of all conversations. . . . his romance certainly interested the professors more than all the reports submitted to the Congress."[22] In 1893, Emmy left Koch and returned to Clausthal. Robert and Emmy Koch were divorced in 1893; Koch married Hedwig Freiberg shortly thereafter. He was fifty, she eighteen. Their marriage was a happy one and lasted through the remainder of his life.

Rivalries developed within the community of scientists who had joined Koch's research institute in Berlin.[23] Emil von Behring, who had joined the Institute in 1889, was an important collaborator of Koch's in studies of tuberculosis. Behring's own studies focused on soluble serum factors in resistance to infection—factors we now recognize as antibodies. Initially making observations on tetanus, Behring then single handedly developed antisera to diphtheria, a life-saving form of therapy. For this work he became the first recipient of the Nobel Prize in Medicine in 1901. Koch felt slighted by the fame that came to Behring and was disappointed when Behring left the institute to work with a pharmaceutical company.

Paul Ehrlich, who was present at Koch's 1882 first presentation of his studies of tuberculosis and who immediately improved upon Koch's staining techniques and who himself suffered from tuberculosis,[24] worked with Behring on diphtheria antiserum. He left Koch's institute in 1896. He and Behring became enemies, Ehrlich feeling that his contributions to the diphtheria research had not been properly recognized. Ehrlich's continued work on immunity was recognized later with a Nobel Prize in 1908.

Koch, now famous throughout the world, received calls to study infectious diseases in many countries. He responded to many of them, studying rinderpest and other diseases of cattle in South Africa and malaria in India and New Guinea. Hedwig accompanied him on several of these expeditions, and both Robert and Hedwig Koch enjoyed life in Africa. In studies of an outbreak of typhoid fever in Germany, Koch was the first to recognize the existence of apparently well persons who were typhoid carriers.

The Nobel Prize was first awarded in 1901, and it immediately became the world's most prestigious medical award. Koch was disappointed when the first award in medicine went to his junior colleague Emil von Behring. He was again disappointed in 1902, when the prize was awarded to Ronald Ross, with whom Koch had worked in Bombay, for identifying the mosquito's role in the transmission of malaria. Finally, in 1905, Koch received his Nobel Prize in Medicine for his studies of tuberculosis.

On October 1, 1904, Koch retired as Director of the Institute for Infectious Diseases in Berlin; his many travels had made him an absentee director for several years. He was 60 years old. In his retirement he and his wife travelled extensively, visiting Africa again, the United States, and Japan. In America, Hedwig, who spoke fluent English, often served as his translator and spokesperson. Koch participated in a major tuberculosis conference held in Washington, D.C. in September 1908. The most controversial topic was tuberculosis in cattle. Although Theobald Smith, an American microbiologist, had established *Mycobacterium bovis* as a separate species distinct from the human organism *Mycobacterium tuberculosis*, Koch and others had argued that the bovine organism was of little importance to humans. The conclusions of the conference emphasized the risk of human infection from contaminated milk, giving new impetus to public health efforts directed towards control of this form of the disease.

Koch returned to Berlin in October 1908. His health began to fail.

He died on May 27, 1910, the victim of a heart attack. His cremated remains rest in a tomb in the Robert Koch Institute for Infectious Diseases.

10

A Distinctly Preventable Disease

New Yorkers may have felt that it took an undue length of time for news of Koch's demonstration of the infectious cause of tuberculosis to reach them (Chapter 9), but they then wasted little time in acting upon the new knowledge. In May 1889, a group of three consultants to the New York City Health Department, led by Hermann Biggs, submitted a report that concluded:

1st. That tuberculosis is a distinctly preventable disease.
2d. That it is not directly inherited; and
3d. That it is acquired by the direct transmission of the tubercle bacillus from the sick to the healthy, usually by means of the dried and pulverized sputum floating as dust through the air.

The measures, then, which are suggested for the prevention of the spread of tuberculosis are:

1st. The security of the public against tubercular meat and milk, attained by a system of rigid official inspection of cattle.
2d. The dissemination among the people of the knowledge that every tubercular person may be an actual source of danger to his associates, . . .
3d. The careful disinfection of rooms and hospital wards that are occupied or have been occupied by phthisical persons."[1]

The Health Department then conducted a survey among physicians and found that nearly all of them felt that no specific public health actions were needed with respect to tuberculosis. Despite this negative response, the Health Department issued in July a circular to health providers

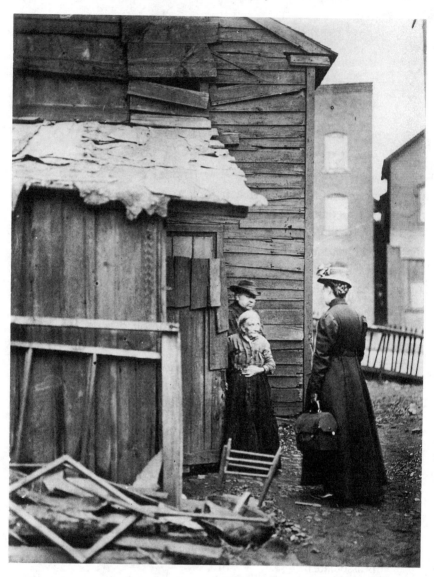

Figure 10.1. A public health nurse visiting a poor family in an urban slum in about 1890. Tuberculosis case finding and health education were important functions of health department nurses. Photograph courtesy of the American Lung Association.

and to the public at large that marked the beginning of a national campaign to rid the American public of the menace of infectious tuberculosis. The tone of this publication foreshadowed the sometimes ludicrous extremes to which this campaign extended. Its injunctions read:

"Rules to be Observed for the Prevention
of the Spread of Consumption

. . . . By observing the following rules the danger of catching the disease will be reduced to a minimum:

I. Do not permit persons having consumption to spit on the floor or on cloths, unless the latter be immediately burned. The expectoration of persons suspected to have consumption should be caught in earthen or glass dishes containing the following solution: Corrosive sublimate,[2] seven grains; water, one pint, and finally thrown into the sewer or burned.

II. Do not sleep in a room occupied by a person who has consumption. The living room of a consumptive patient should have as little furniture as practicable. Hangings should be carefully avoided. The use of carpets and rugs ought always to be avoided.

III. Do not fail to wash thoroughly the eating utensils of a person who has consumption as soon after eating as possible, using boiling water for the purpose.

IV. Do not mingle the unwashed clothing of a consumptive person with similar clothing of other persons. The soiled clothing of a consumptive person should be removed at once, put in boiling water for forty-five minutes, or otherwise disinfected.

V. Do not fail to catch the bowel discharges of a consumptive person with diarrhea in a vessel containing corrosive sublimate seven grains to water one pint.

VI. Do not fail to consult the family physician regarding the social relations of persons suffering from suspected consumption.

VII. Do not permit mothers suspected of having consumption to nurse their offspring.

VIII. Household pets (animals or birds) are quite susceptible to tuberculosis,[3] therefore, do not expose them to persons afflicted with consumption; also, do not keep but destroy at once all household pets suspected of having consumption, otherwise they may give it to human beings.

IX. Do not fail to cleanse thoroughly the floors, walls and ceilings of the living and sleeping rooms of persons suffering from consumption at least once in two weeks.[4]

Chopin would have been no more welcome in New York City in 1889 than he was in Mallorca and Barcelona forty years earlier!

We now know, as will be seen, that tuberculosis is spread almost exclusively by dried tubercle bacilli coughed into the air. Once deposited on floors and other surfaces, these germs do not have wings, jet engines, catapults, or other means of launching themselves into the atmosphere. Thus, by today's standards, the caution against sleeping in the same room as a tuberculous patient makes sense, but almost all of the rest of the actions recommended to the people of New York do not. However, the idea that something could be done to prevent the spread of tuberculous infection was an exciting one, and few would argue against taking action.

But some did argue against it. Only a few years earlier, on January 12, 1894, the American College of Physicians, a prestigious group then and now, passed a remarkable resolution opposing compulsory notification by physicians of health departments of cases of tuberculosis. Sir William Osler, the country's most famous physician at the time, argued against the resolution. But other voices prevailed. Dr. Owen J. Wister argued, "those of us who are not in the intimate confidence of Nature find it difficult to understand how a hereditary disease can be eradicated by measures which only limit its spread by contagion; and if it is not hereditary, whence come those forms of tuberculosis other than pulmonary? It cannot be pretended that babies a year or two old get tubercular meningitis by contagion, nor can white swelling, nor suppurating glands nor the many other exhibitions of scrofula come from contagion."[5] Dr. Wister may have been a member of a prestigious medical society, but he clearly did not understand the work of Villemin and Koch!

As fervor for preventing the transmission of tuberculosis spread across North America and Europe, many public health regulations and actions were implemented. Common drinking cups were outlawed on railroads. In France and England, children were removed from their homes to be boarded out when a parent developed the disease. Patients in tuberculosis hospitals had letters to their family sterilized in steam autoclaves before being mailed, a treatment that surely made them not only sterile but illegible. Spitting became a focus of public attention. Plain clothes police officers were assigned to arrest public spitters. The

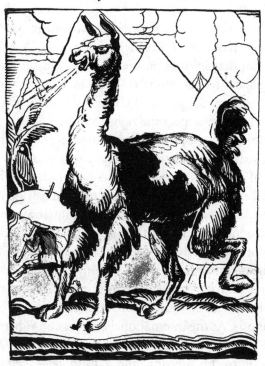

When A Llama Gets Sore
He Spits!
He's the world's best spitter
but
Who **Wants to be a Llama?**

Figure 10.2. The first page of a two-page circular distributed by the National Tuberculosis Association as a part of its anti-spitting campaign. Courtesy of the American Lung Association.

Rochester, New York Public Health Association printed slips that its members could pass out to offenders. They read, "MY FRIEND. Let me remind you that spitting on the sidewalks, in the street cars, or in any public place is forbidden by law. It is unsanitary and a menace to the health of others. It spreads TUBERCULOSIS. Every gentleman will obey the law and respect the rights of others."[6]

The champions of public health measures for the control of tuberculosis also turned their legislative and regulatory weapons on tuberculosis in dairy and meat cattle. The American bacteriologist Theobald Smith demonstrated in 1896 that the bovine tuberculosis germ, *Mycobacterium bovis*, is separate and distinct from the human strain of the organism. Alone among scientists of the day, but riding on his unimpeachable reputation, Robert Koch declared that the bovine organism did not cause disease in humans. He was wrong, as others had already recognized. But others overemphasized the importance of the bovine strain; it probably never caused more than about ten percent of cases of human tuberculosis. At the international congress on tuberculosis held in Washington in 1908, Koch defended his views initially. The press gave much attention to this meeting, and a *Washington Post* headline read, "Koch Stands Fast." But at the end, Koch did not object to the conferences recommendations for public health campaigns to control tuberculosis in cows. Meanwhile, these campaigns had already been launched in North America and Europe. Certification and pasteurization of milk became the norm. Koch's tuberculin came into use for the diagnosis of bovine tuberculosis even earlier than it did for recognizing human disease, and infected cattle were slaughtered. Today, while sporadic cases of bovine disease occur, this form of tuberculosis is no longer a problem in North America and western Europe.[7]

Common sense and scientific knowledge about the transmission of tuberculosis finally caught up with corrosive sublimate and leaflets against spitting. In fact, the concept of airborne transmission of tuberculous infection was embraced by many workers in the first two decades following Koch's discovery of the tubercle bacillus. Koch himself did experiments in which animals were infected with aerosol sprays of tuberculosis germs.[8] However, it was the work of William Firth Wells in the 1930s and 1940s and of Richard L. Riley (who had been a tuberculosis patient himself) in the 1950s and 1960s that firmly established our present knowledge of how tuberculosis is spread through the air. Their work culminated in studies conducted by Riley, Wells, and their collaborators in Baltimore. They established a study center adjacent to a six room tuberculosis ward, and for two years the air from these rooms was evacuated through a chamber containing cages for guinea pigs. Thus, they were able to study the infectiousness of the air from the environment of these patients. Seventy-one of one hundred and fifty-six exposed guinea pigs became infected, an average of three each month. Two of sixty-two patients in the tuberculosis ward contributed the infections of nineteen of these animals. Some patients did not infect any guinea pigs. Breathing the air surrounding infectious tuberculosis patients was clearly established as a route to infection.[9]

When a person with tuberculosis coughs—or talks or sings—the moist breath expelled contains tiny droplets of water. Bacteria may reside at the core of some of these droplets. Within a foot or two of the person's mouth, the moisture of these tiny droplets evaporates, sometimes leaving a dried droplet nucleus suspended in the air. If these droplet nuclei contain virulent tubercle bacilli, they are then infectious particles. Because they are so light, they may remain suspended in the air for many hours. Because they are so small, they reach deep into the lungs when they are inhaled by an uninfected person. Because they are so virulent, they easily establish a focus of tuberculous infection. These facts have led to a modern emphasis on ventilation in the control of tuberculosis. Tubercle bacilli are easily killed by ultraviolet light, including that of ordinary daylight, and thus modern isolation facilities rely on evacuation of air to the outside.

Frequency of cough, number of tubercle bacilli in sputum, and extent of disease are all factors that have been identified as making some individual patients more infectious than others. These factors are not surprises, for they are features of tuberculosis that lead to the expelling of greater numbers of tubercle bacilli.

What happened to concerns about the tuberculous patient's bedding, clothing, and personal effects? What of white washing the walls of a patient's room, as Chopin's Barcelona innkeeper was required to do? What of corrosive sublimate? A series of investigations of outbreaks of tuberculosis during the middle part of the twentieth century made it increasingly obvious that it is only the air—no other part of the environment—

that poses an infectious hazard. One of the earliest and most elegant of these studies was an investigation by T.V. Hyge of a large outbreak in a Danish school. Early in 1942, seventy of one hundred and five previously uninfected students were found to have become infected with tubercle bacilli. The infections were traced to a single classroom used by a teacher who was found to have tuberculosis in both lungs. The room was in the basement of the school (it was used as an air raid shelter during the war), and was both dark and poorly ventilated. Students who used the class room early in the day before the diseased teacher taught in it did not become infected; students who used the room later in the day after the teacher was there did. Overnight, with ventilation and settling of particles in the air, the room became safe once more.[10] Other similar studies of outbreaks followed. In 1964, John Chapman and Margaret Dyerly reported a study of tuberculosis in the children of patients hospitalized with tuberculosis in Dallas, Texas. Although no special effort was made to clean the houses from which the tuberculosis patients came, not a one of sixty-two previously uninfected, susceptible children became infected after the parent was hospitalized. No risk of tuberculosis transmission remained behind in the home.[11]

In 1967, an expert committee of the National Tuberculosis Association concluded that covering of the nose and mouth by patients while coughing, good ventilation of patient rooms, and sterilization of air with ultraviolet light if rooms could not be ventilated or if air was to be recirculated should be the cornerstones of tuberculosis infection control. "The aim of decontamination", the report stated, "is to remove . . . any tubercle bacilli excreted by the patients into the air."[12] These principles still apply. A recent requirement of the Occupational Safety and Health Administration that health care workers exposed to tuberculosis patients wear high efficiency aerosol particulate respirators sparked a storm of protest from the medical community because this approach ignores the now well established effectiveness of ventilation, impedes care of patients unnecessarily, requires the wearing of uncomfortable devices that are expensive, and has not been studied for effectiveness in preventing the spread of tuberculosis.

Tuberculosis continues to occur in all parts of the world. In developing countries, most transmission of infection probably happens at night when all members of a family sleep in a single, poorly ventilated room.

In North America and Europe, custodial institutions, homeless shelters, and other closed environments are often the loci of outbreaks. As we saw in Chapter 3, St. Francis of Assisi may have contracted his infection while in prison. Today's prisons may not be much safer.

In 1992, a homeless man in Minneapolis, Minnesota presented to Hennepin County Medical Center with a six-month-long illness characterized by fever, cough, weakness, and a weight loss of more than more than sixty-five pounds.[13] He was found to have pulmonary tuberculosis with large numbers of tuberculosis germs in his sputum. As his illness had progressed, he had spent most of his time in a neighborhood bar. The local health department began an investigation. Ninety-seven persons were identified among the bar workers and regular patrons who were contacts of this infectious man. Among them, thirty-nine were found to be infected with tubercle bacilli, and fourteen persons either already had or soon developed clinical tuberculosis. Six additional related cases developed, two in persons who had never been in the bar but were infected by others who had caught their disease there. Thus, one man in the closed environment of the neighborhood bar spread his infection to dozens of others and caused illness in twenty persons.

In 1993, a college student in Maryland with unrecognized tuberculosis infected approximately eighty of her classmates and four young children in families of friends with tubercle bacilli. Among her eight dormitory suite-mates, she infected six. Six of the infected college students and all four of the young children developed active tuberculosis. All of them recovered with treatment.[14]

In 1993 the local health department was notified of a case of tuberculosis in an office worker in Melbourne, Australia. Five months later a second case was reported from the same office. An investigation was launched, and it was found that one-fourth of two hundred and ten workers in the same office had been infected with tubercle bacilli.[15]

Several recent episodes of the spread of tuberculous infection among passengers and crew of modern jet aircraft have been studied and described in medical journals.[16] Some of these aircraft recirculate cabin air, others do not. However, recirculated air is passed through high efficiency filters that remove all bacteria. Air flow in aircraft cabins is high. What is the problem? The unsurmountable difficulty is the high density of passenger seating in a small volume, cigar-shaped aircraft cabin.

No matter how high the air flow, passengers sitting near infectious persons are likely to be exposed.

Whether in a bar, a school, an office, or an airplane, tuberculosis remains an infectious disease. Despite great technological advances, there remains a need for both vigilance and common sense in combatting its further spread.

11

Heroes

A young nurse was in charge of a general medical ward. Her nursing station, where she worked each day, was centrally located in the ward. Air from the ward was evacuated by the ventilation system through an exhaust duct opening just above her desk. Thus, all of the air from the ward passed through her work station on its way to the outside. She developed tuberculosis, recovering only after many months of drug treatment.

A laboratory technician worked on a project testing the efficacy of a sterilizing device for removing live tuberculosis germs from the air. She was assigned to operate an aerosol unit—an atomizer—that produced a mist of tuberculosis germs in front of the air sterilizing device. She developed tuberculosis, from which she ultimately recovered, but not before she had suffered extensive damage to one of her lungs.

A medical resident participated in the attempted resuscitation of an elderly man who died within an hour of entering the hospital. Nothing was known of the medical history of the man, to whom the resident gave mouth-to-mouth respiration. At autopsy, the man proved to have extensive tuberculosis. The resident developed tuberculosis, and infected one of the interns working with him before he was made noninfectious by drug treatment.

A physician had a routine chest Xray examination, which showed tuberculosis. On investigation, the disease proved to be due to a strain of tubercle bacilli resistant to most of the standard curative drugs for this disease. Epidemiologic investigation established that the physician had become infected several years earlier during internship, caring for hospitalized patients. The source patient was not identified. Ultimately, after surgery to remove infected tissue and a course of treatment with alternative drugs, the physician recovered.

These four vignettes are all true.[1] The nurse, the doctors, the laboratory technician all suffered tuberculosis because they did what they were trained to do in the care of the sick. None of them questioned their actions, not at the time, not later after suffering major illness. They were all treated effectively, and are all alive and well now, but this happy outcome does not diminish their heroism.

During the first half of this century, when tuberculosis was a life-threatening disease for which curative treatment did not exist, four out of ten medical and nursing students became infected with the germs of tuberculosis during their training years.[2] About one in twenty developed active disease. This was the accepted cost of a life of service in health care. But this cost, known to all, did not stop young men and women from dedicating their lives to the care of the sick. Today, our knowledge of the infectious nature of tuberculosis and the mode of its spread allows health care workers to provide medical care in relative safety, although the four victims described above all acquired their disease in modern times.

The history of tuberculosis contains the stories of many physicians who themselves suffered from the disease—Laennec, Ehrlich, Flick, Trudeau, Frost, Lurie, Myers, and many others. Less heralded are thousands of others who also suffered from the ravages of tuberculosis. They who fought to conquer the greatest of the infectious diseases to afflict the human race and they who gave of themselves to minister to its victims are the heroes of one of the noblest battles the world has seen.

PART III

Of Languor and Lymphocytes
Susceptibility and Resistance to Tuberculosis

Even though I walk through the valley of the shadow of death, I fear no evil; . . .

Psalm 23:4[1]

I have a little shadow that goes in and out with me,
And what can be the use of him is more than I can see.

A Child's Garden of Verses
Robert Louis Stevenson[2]

Two Men of Letters

John Keats and Robert Louis Stevenson both had tuberculosis. The course of the illness was strikingly different in the two writers, and the difference dramatically highlights the importance that resistance and susceptibility to the disease play in the course and pathogenesis of tuberculosis.

John Keats was born in London in October 1795.[3] His father, an innkeeper, died after falling off a horse when Keats was still a boy. His mother remarried, but this second marriage did not last more than a few months, and the Keats family moved to live with her parents. John was sent to the school of John Clarke at Enfield, a relatively progressive school that emphasized not simply the classics but also natural and physical sciences; Clarke was a friend of Joseph Priestly, England's preeminent scientist of the day. Keats was a bright and diligent student and an avid reader. Short of stature, he was active and sometimes feisty. He enjoyed sports. Some biographers speak of him as an amateur boxer; others simply note that he was quick to become involved in boyhood scraps and fights. By all accounts, he was a happy and active youth and in vigorous good health.

When Keats was fourteen years old, his mother died of tuberculosis. During her final illness, Keats left school and devoted much of his time to her, sitting with her, reading to her, giving her medicines, feeding her, often spending entire nights at her bedside. Following her death, Keats became the ward of his grandfather, who arranged for Keats to be apprenticed to Mr. Thomas Hammond, a respected and accomplished surgeon, so that Keats might begin the study of medicine. Some have suggested that Keats was coerced into this apprenticeship, but it is much more likely that he was strongly attracted to a career as a physician and that he entered upon his apprenticeship with enthusiasm. Keats was fourteen or fifteen—there are conflicting data—when he began his apprenticeship. He lived in quarters provided by his mentor, followed him on his daily rounds, and learned the rudiments of pulling teeth, setting broken bones, and dressing wounds. These were the principal skills of surgeons of that era. Keats enjoyed the work, and the four or five years he spent with Hammond were happy, busy, and healthy ones.

In the summer of 1815, Keats entered Guys Hospital Medical School, to this day a distinguished London medical school. A year of hospital medical school training following five apprenticeship years was the usual course of medical training at that time and the minimum requirement for the recently established licensure by the Apothecaries Society. In October, he was assigned as a dresser to Mr. William Lucks, a surgeon at Guys Hospital who was not held in high regard by his peers and did not serve Keats well as a role model. The position of dresser was that of an assistant, and Keats did gain valuable experience in caring for Lucks' patients. Guys Hospital offered many lectures and demonstrations by the most distinguished physicians of the day, and Keats was particularly influenced by Mr. Astley Cooper, an eminent surgeon.

Keats did well as a medical student, and on July 25, 1816 he passed the licensing examination on his first attempt, apparently with ease. Many of his fellow students required more than one attempt to pass this rigorous examination. Because he had not yet attained the minimum age of twenty-one, Keats had to wait several months to be licensed, and he remained a dresser at Guys Hospital until March of 1817.

During his year at Guys Hospital, Keats began to write poetry, and his poetry was well received by other literary persons in London, if not always by critics. In the chemistry notebook of one of his classmates he penned, "A thing of beauty is a constant joy." This line was later changed to become the famous opening line of *Endymion*, which was finished shortly after Keats left Guys Hospital—"A thing of beauty is a joy forever." Keats' ode, *On First Looking into Chapman's Homer*, was composed three months after he passed his qualifying examination.

As the hospital year progressed, Keats became less and less certain that he wished to be a physician, and before it ended he had determined not to practice medicine. There has been much written about Keats' state of mind and the various factors that might have influenced his decision. For whatever reason, Keats decided that he would rather be a poet than a physician. Although, he never practiced the profession for which he had trained and become licensed, Keats did not regret the training. On May 3, 1818, he wrote in a letter, "Were I to study physic or rather Medicine again, I feel it would not make the least difference to my Poetry; when the mind is in its infancy a Bias is in reality a Bias, but when we have acquired more strength, a Bias becomes no Bias. Every department of Knowledge we see excellent and calculated towards a great whole. I am so convinced of this, that I am glad at not having given away my medical Books. . . . An extensive knowledge is needful to thinking people—it takes away the heat and fever; and helps, by widening speculation, to ease the Burden of the Mystery."[4]

Keats left Guys Hospital to live with his brothers George and Tom in Well Walk, Hampstead. Shortly thereafter, George married and emigrated to America. With Tom, John Keats led an active life, writing poetry and walking, taking long treks in the British Midlands, Lake District, and Scotland. He was in excellent health. His brother Tom, however, began to suffer illness, and in August 1818 it was apparent that Tom, as his mother before him, was to be a victim of tuberculosis. Keats remained with his brother at Well Walk, caring for him until he died on December 1, 1818.

Short of money, Keats again contemplated practicing surgery, but he did not do so. He moved a number of times, often living with friends, of which he had many. Charles Brown and Joseph Severn were particularly good comrades, and he continued his walks with them. He was active and in good health. He wrote prolifically. In fact, almost all of his best work was written during a period of about one year, from early 1819 to early 1820. In May 1819 he completed his *Ode on a Grecian Urn*, with its famous romantic couplet:

"'Beauty is truth, truth beauty'—that is all
Ye know on earth, and all ye need to know."

Keats was attracted to a number of young women, and in December 1819 (romantic legend says on Christmas day) after a year of courtship, he became engaged to Fanny Brawne.

On February 3, 1820, John Keats coughed up blood. This first sign of his tuberculosis was an event that has been described by many biographers. He was climbing into bed, and spit blood onto the sheet. At the time he was staying with Charles Brown in London, and he said to his friend, "Bring me the candle, Brown; and let me see this blood." After examining the expectoration he said, "I know the colour of that blood;—it is arterial blood;—I cannot be deceived in that colour; that drop of blood is my death-warrant. I must die."[5] Surely Keats, at that moment, made his own diagnosis and understood its import. This sudden onset of disease came against a background of health. During the preceding year, Keats had complained of frequent sore throats, but while this symptom may have many causes, tuberculosis is rarely among them.

Keats' friend Brown called a local surgeon to see the sick poet. This doctor withdrew blood from Keats—bleeding to remove evil humors was then a widely used therapy for many illnesses—and prescribed bed rest and a restricted diet. Confining Keats to his room, the illness forced a separation from his beloved Fanny. Keats continued to cough up blood from time to time, and on March 8, 1820 he was seen by Dr. Robert Bree. Bree was a noted physician, an expert on tuberculosis, and the owner of one of the few stethoscopes in England. This instrument had been invented by Laennec in France the year before. Bree used it to examine Keats' chest, and then reassured Keats that his troubles were due to indigestion and that he was not suffering from tuberculosis. He urged Keats to get out of bed, and within two days Keats was again up and walking.

Did the respected Dr. Bree fail to recognize the nature of Keats' illness? Probably not. It is more likely that Bree sought to comfort his patient and saw little use in giving him the diagnosis of a disease for which no effective treatment existed. Today we emphasize accuracy of communication between doctor and patient. Then, diagnoses were often not disclosed so as to provide greater peace of mind to patients.

Keats was not deceived. He took several short sea voyages, widely thought to be effective in the treatment of tuberculosis, but found himself too weak to sustain lengthy trips. During the summer of 1820, he again took pen to hand, and he also resumed his relationship with Fanny Brawne, spending time with her and her family. Although he wrote, he never produced work of the quality of his earlier efforts. In fact, Keats, once suddenly taken ill, never again regained good health. He appears to have been defeated in both mind and body from the onset of his illness.

Percy Bysshe Shelley was Keats' contemporary, friend and admirer, and equally famous as a romantic poet. Shelley, who often anticipated death in his poems, also had tuberculosis. When he learned of Keats' illness, he wrote to his friend:

"My Dear Keats:

"I hear with great pain the dangerous accident you have undergone and Mr. Gisborne, who gives me the account of it, adds that you continue to wear a consumptive appearance. This consumption is a disease particularly fond of people who write such good verse as you have done, and with the assistance of an English winter it can often indulge the selection. I do not think that young and amiable poets are at all bound to gratify its taste; they have entered into no bond with the muses to that effect."[6]

Reluctantly and perhaps fearfully, Keats acceded to the advice of his physicians and friends and determined to go to Italy. The sea voyage would be good for his health, and Italy provided a favorable climate for consumptive patients. Dr. James Clark, physician to Queen Victoria and to many literary figures of the era and a man with a well established reputation for treating tuberculosis,[7] had taken up residence in Rome, and a voyage to Italy would provide Keats with the opportunity to consult with him.

Accompanied by his friend, Joseph Severn, and taking with him a lock of his beloved Fanny's hair, Keats boarded the *Maria Crowther* on September 17, 1820 and sailed for Italy the following day. There were two other passengers on the vessel, a Miss Cotterell, who also suffered from tuberculosis, and a Mrs. Pidgeon, who accompanied her. The small ship was soon beset by storms, and Keats, barely able to move about, found himself attending to the sea sickness of his fellow passengers. After ten days beating unsuccessfully into unfavorable winds, the *Maria Crowther* put into Portsmouth to wait out the storm. The weather improved, and the ship again sailed for Italy. The passage was marked by more bad weather, and Keats became weaker during the trip. He had further episodes of hemoptysis—coughing of blood. The vessel reached

Naples on October 21, but Keats was forced to remain on board during a ten day quarantine period.

Finally ashore, Keats travelled to Rome, where he saw Dr. Clark. On November 30, he wrote to his friend Charles Brown, "Dr. Clark is very attentive to me; he says there is very little the matter with my lungs, but my stomach, he says, is very bad." Once again, there was an effort to shield Keats from his ominous diagnosis. Clark prescribed gentle horseback rides and arranged housing for Keats at his own expense. Ten days later Keats had a massive hemoptysis. Clark phlebotomized him and put him on restricted diet. On December 13, Clark wrote, "Poor fellow, he is now so ill as to be constantly confined to bed, . . . the affection of his lungs increasing and the state of his mind is the most deplorable possible. . . . recovery is almost out of the question."[8]

The end was near. Cared for by his friend Joseph Severn, Keats was unable to get out of bed, and he grew steadily weaker. Severn wrote to the Brawne family on January 11 that Keats "had changed to calmness and quietude," now accepting of his coming death.[9] He was racked by cough. For long hours he slept or was only semiconscious. On Friday afternoon, February 23, 1821, he called to Severn, "Severn, lift me up, for I am dying. I shall die easy. . . . Don't be frightened. Thank God it has come."[10] Those were his last words. Shortly before midnight he passed quietly from life.

So it was that John Keats was stricken when in robust good health to fall victim in eleven months' time to unrelenting tuberculosis. The story of Robert Louis Stevenson contrasts so remarkably with that of Keats that one would hardly think that they both suffered from the same disease.

Robert Louis Balfour Stevenson was born in Edinburgh, Scotland on November 13, 1850, nearly three decades after Keats' death. An only child, he was the son of a dour Calvinist lighthouse builder. If his father was stern and melancholic, his mother was cheerful, intelligent, and interested in literature. She encouraged the penchants for reading and for writing stories that appeared early in her son.

Stevenson was chronically ill as a child. He probably developed tuberculosis as a boy.[11] His schooling was frequently interrupted, and he was repeatedly taken to the sea shore for his health. Some biographers believe that his mother had tuberculosis, and her father before her. Stevenson was a young man of twenty-three when he first was told he might have tuberculosis. He was seen at that time by a London special-ist, Dr. Andrew Clark, who made a diagnosis of threatening phthisis. Dr. Clark felt that Stevenson suffered from nervous exhaustion and rec-ommended that he spend the coming winter on the Riviera.

Following Dr. Clark's advice, Stevenson spent the winter of 1873 in Mentone near Monte Carlo. He became deeply depressed and preoccu-pied with death, which he felt would be soon to come. But by Decem-ber, his health was improving and his depression lifted. He returned to Scotland in the spring and began to study law in Edinburgh. He passed the examinations and was admitted to the bar in July 1875, but he never practiced law. Over the next few years, Stevenson returned to southern France often, finding that the warmer climate was beneficial to his health. In Grez, France he met Fanny Van de Grift Osborne, an unhappily married American woman with two children, ten years Stevenson's senior, who had gone to France while her divorce proceed-ings were in progress. Stevenson and Fanny Osborne fell in love.

Against the advice of his friends and without telling his parents, Stevenson pursued Fanny following her return to California. Stevenson initially camped in the countryside near Monterrey, a life style widely thought to benefit tuberculosis.[12] Stevenson married Fanny on May 19, 1880, but ill health—fever, night sweats, and cough—typical symp-toms of tuberculosis—pursued him, and the couple returned to Edin-burgh. There Stevenson consulted his uncle, Dr. George Balfour, who had no doubt about the cause of his ill health. He had tuberculosis, and he should go to the Alps. Stevenson again consulted Dr. Andrew Clark in London, and Clark confirmed the diagnosis. In November 1880, Stevenson, accompanied by Fanny, went to Davos, Switzerland, the fa-mous alpine spa that later provided the setting for Thomas Mann's clas-sic novel, *The Magic Mountain.*

Life in Davos suited Stevenson, and his condition steadily improved. He was allowed to write for three hours daily by his physician, Dr. Ruedi. He wrote most of *Treasure Island* at Davos, and in April 1882 he was well enough so that Dr. Ruedi gave him permission to return to the flat land below. Back in Edinburgh, Stevenson soon became ill again, and in July he had a major pulmonary hemorrhage. He again sought advice from Dr. Clark, who again advised him to go to southern France. Stevenson and Fanny settled near Marseilles. *Treasure Island* was published and was immediately successful; indeed this book has never been out of print since. Royalty payments arrived regularly. However, Stevenson's illness continued, with recurrent bleeding from his diseased lungs. His physicians strapped his right arm to his chest to splint his chest during breathing, and Stevenson was forced to write using his left hand. During one desperate episode, he took paper and wrote, "if this is death, it is an easy one."

The next year saw the return of relatively good health, and during the three year interval from 1884 to the summer of 1887 Stevenson was well, living in Bournemouth, near London, and writing actively. *Dr. Jekyll and Mr. Hyde* and *Kidnapped* were finished and sent to the publisher. *A Child's Garden of Verse* was completed at this time. He had worked on this collection of light-hearted children's poems for several years, dashing off many of them quickly. The couplet about his shadow, which is quoted at the beginning of this section of this book (page 99), can be read to reflect on Stevenson's chronic illness as a child, but the rest of the poem puts it in a context of frivolity, not misery. During this time, Stevenson came to think of himself as a story teller, a pied piper playing tunes on a penny whistle. Later, his Samoan friends would call him Tusitala, a story teller.

In the summer of 1887, Stevenson's chronic and relapsing tuberculosis recurred once again, with additional hemorrhages from his lungs. He again saw Dr. Clark and also consulted a Dr. Scott, a Bournemouth physician whom he had come to trust. Both doctors agreed that his tuberculosis was progressing, and they recommended that Stevenson try the climate of Colorado. And so, on August 22, 1887, Robert Louis Stevenson once again set off on a voyage seeking a place that would prove favorable for the return of his health. He was accompanied not only by his wife, Fanny, but also by his mother.

On arrival in New York City, Stevenson, now a famous author, was welcomed and lionized by social and literary figures. He and Fanny enjoyed New York. Ultimately, they decided against Colorado and went to Saranac Lake. Saranac Lake had become famous as a treatment center for tuberculosis, and Edward Livingston Trudeau's Adirondack Cottage Sanitarium had become famous. Trudeau was widely known and respected for his skill in treating tuberculosis, especially among the socially prominent people whom Stevenson met in New York.

Stevenson took up residence in the Baker Cottage of Trudeau's sanatorium for the winter of 1887-88. He and Trudeau did not initially find themselves compatible, but by the end of Stevenson's stay in the Adirondacks, they were good friends. Nor did Stevenson fit in well with the local townspeople. He did not fish and he did not hunt, favorite local activities. He did enjoy ice skating. An incessant cigarette smoker, he spent long hours in solitude. His stories written during his Saranac winter included *The Master of Ballantrae*, *The Wrong Box*, and *A Christmas Sermon*. Stevenson wrote to a friend, "We are high up in the Adirondack Mountains living in a guide's cottage in the most primitive fashion. The maid does the cooking (we have little beyond venison and bread to cook) and the boy comes every morning to carry water from a distant spring for drinking purposes. It is already very cold, but we have caulked the doors and windows as one caulks a boat, and have laid in a store of extraordinary garments made by the Canadian Indians. . . . It is something like Davos here."

Years later, after Stevenson's death in Samoa, Trudeau was quoted as saying, "He did not die of tuberculosis, as I made it a point of finding out. . . . Yet it is a mistake to say that he never had tuberculosis. Although, while I took care of him, he had none of the active symptoms, such as hemorrhage, or fever, or tubercle bacilli, present, yet he undoubtedly had had tuberculosis. It may have become active again after he left Saranac, so there is no telling just how much that disease may have contributed to his mortal illness in Samoa."[13] Perhaps reflecting Trudeau's statement that he had none of the active signs of tuberculosis while at Saranac, a number of biographers have questioned the nature of Stevenson's illness. Although it is possible to think of other illnesses that might have produced the disease picture seen in Stevenson, none is likely, and tuberculosis today seems to be the almost certain diagnosis for the famous author. It should be remembered that radiologic examinations were not available during Stevenson's life time and that stains to identify tubercle bacilli had first been described by Koch only five years before Stevenson placed himself under Trudeau's care. Trudeau learned the technique of staining tubercle bacilli in 1885, only two years before Stevenson's arrival in Saranac Lake.[14] If he tried to identify tubercle bacilli in Stevenson's sputum, it must have been one of Trudeau's early attempts at doing so, and the techniques available at that time were much more crude and technically difficult than they are today.

April 1888 found Stevenson well and travelling again—first to California, but for only two weeks—then on by ship to the South Pacific. He stopped in Hawaii, where he visited Father Damien's leper colony on Molokai. In Hawaii, illness overcame him again, with more bleeding from his lungs. He then went to Samoa, where he took up residence on a four hundred acre plantation. He enjoyed life on the island where he was to spend the rest of his life. Although he was generally healthy, there were also times of illness. In 1893, he wrote to a friend, "For fourteen years I have not had a day's real health; I have wakened sick and gone to bed weary; and I have done my work unflinchingly. I have written in bed, and written out of it, written in hemorrhages, written in sickness, written torn by coughing, written when my head swam for weakness; and for so long, it seems to me I have won my wager and recovered my glove. I am better now, have been, rightly speaking, since first I came to the pacific; and still, few are the days when I am not in some physical distress. And the battle goes on—ill or well, is a trifle; so as it goes."[15]

The end of Robert Louis Stevenson's life came suddenly on December 3, 1894. He was in good health and high spirits, serving wine to his wife and friends on the veranda of his Samoan home while supper was being prepared. Suddenly, he put both hands to his head and called to Fanny, "What's that? Do I look strange?" He fell to the floor unconscious, and died quietly several hours later. The diagnosis of the local physicians who attended him was cerebral apoplexy. Viewed from the perspective of modern medicine, it seems likely that his massive and abrupt stroke might have been caused by rupture of an aneurysm of a cerebral artery. After a life of chronic and relapsing illness, a life of happiness and sorrow, a life never out of the umbra of tuberculosis, a life spent traveling in search of a cure, a life of enormous literary productivity, Robert Louis Stevenson, one of the most prolific story tellers of all times, died of a cause not related to his tuberculosis.

Both John Keats and Robert Louis Stevenson suffered from tuberculosis, and we must now turn our attention to understanding something of the disease that could have produced such different courses of illness in two persons. In medical terms, we must now try to understand the pathogenesis of tuberculosis—in ordinary language, the process by which the tubercle bacillus causes sickness and sometimes death. Unfortunately, we can more easily recount what may or may not happen than we can explain why or why not.

When the tuberculosis germ spreads through the air from an infectious patient to its next victim, it takes up residence in the lungs of the unfortunate person who inhales it. But the victim is not defenseless, and very promptly the cellular defenders of the lung—scavenger cells called macrophages—swallow up the invading tubercle bacillus in the same fashion that they by their nature are prepared to ingest any microscopic-sized invader. A nonspecific inflammatory response is then mounted, and the newly infected human host to tubercle bacilli is usually no more aware of what has happened than is one who inhales a speck of dust. The chance of this primary infection event occurring for any single person is determined by luck and the circumstances in which the person lives. The Brontë children, dwelling in a house in which all others had tuberculosis, had little hope of escaping infection with tuberculosis germs; most children in North America and Europe today have almost no opportunity to meet this germ. What happens next—or rather what sometimes does and sometimes does not happen next—is uniquely characteristic of tuberculosis, and the way in which it happens and the reasons that subsequent events transpire or do not transpire remain to this day some of the great mysteries of medical science.

Of those infected with tuberculosis germs, approximately five to eight percent are destined to develop disease from these germs. The immune mechanisms that mediate host resistance completely protect the other ninety-two to ninety-five percent, although the tubercle bacilli may remain alive in their tissues throughout the rest of their lives. For some individuals—Eleanor Roosevelt is a good example—mechanisms of resistance offer protection for decades, only to fail at some late time with disease then resulting from germs acquired scores of years previously. Many factors appear to play a role in deciding whether a person will fall in the five to eight percent due to be victims and when it will happen. Certainly heredity plays a role, and so also do nutrition and other aspects of general health. Among those in whom tuberculosis does develop, other factors influence the course and severity of disease. Among the known factors, age is obviously important. Infants are very susceptible, school-aged children very resistant, adolescents and young adults—especially young women—again susceptible, and older adults resistant until they approach their senescent years.[16] Many other factors, including immune status and coexistent diseases, confound this picture. Finally, just as Keats and Stevenson suffered very differently from the assaults of the same microbial enemy, the clinical course of tuberculosis varies enormously from patient to patient, and we do not understand why.

Keats and Stevenson—two men of letters, two persons afflicted with tuberculosis—represent opposite poles on the sphere of resistance to tuberculosis. Keats was seized from a life of vigor and destroyed by the relentless advance of his adversary from the moment of first affliction. He lived less than one year after becoming ill. Stevenson struggled on, never conquered, never conquering, always productive despite the shadow that went in and out with him for three decades or more.

John Keats was buried in Italy in a grave marked only by daisies and violets. Robert Louis Stevenson was laid to rest on a South Pacific hillside, his tombstone inscribed with the epitaph he had written:

> Under the wide and starry sky,
> Dig the grave and let me lie,
> Glad did I live and gladly die,
> And I laid me down with a will.
> This be the verse you grave for me;
> Here he lies where he longed to be;
> Home is the sailor, home from the sea,
> And the hunter home from the hill.

13

A Brownish Transparent Liquid

On August 3, 1890, Robert Koch, whose life and pioneering work are described in Chapter 9, addressed the Tenth International Medical Congress in Berlin. He was honored by the invitation to speak, and his audience expected that he might use this occasion to announce yet another dramatic discovery. Could one expect less of the renowned Dr. Koch? Koch chose as his topic "Ueber bakteriologische Forschung"— On Bacteriological Research. His rambling presentation reviewed recent advances in the new science of bacteriology, emphasizing his own contributions. He then approached the conclusion of his remarks with the following electrifying words:

". . . . I continued the quest and I ultimately found substances that halted the growth of tuberculosis bacilli not only in test tubes but also in animal bodies. As everyone who experiments with tuberculosis finds, investigations of the disease are very slow; mine are no exception. Thus, although I have been occupied with these attempts for nearly one year, my study of these substances is not yet complete. I can only communicate that guinea pigs, which are known to be particularly susceptible to tuberculosis, if subjected to the operation of such substances, no longer react when injected with tuberculosis bacilli, and that in guinea pigs in which tuberculosis has already reached an advanced stage, the disease can be completely halted without otherwise harming the body.

"At this time I conclude only that it is possible to render harmless the pathogenic bacteria that are found in a living body and to do this without disadvantage to the body. Previously, this possibility had been questioned.

"However the further hopes associated with these attempts may be fulfilled—it may be possible, given a bacterial infectious disease, to master the microscopic yet previously uncontrollable invaders within the human body. . . ."[1]

On November 15, 1890, pressured by the enormous clamor that followed his dramatic announcement that the world's greatest scourge could be "completely halted without otherwise harming the body," Koch published a further description of his remedy.[2] He described it at this time as "a brownish transparent liquid" to be freshly diluted and injected into tuberculous patients. In fact, what Koch had done was to kill broth cultures of tubercle bacilli by boiling, remove the dead bacteria by filtration, and then concentrate this "tuberculin" ten-fold by evaporation.

Koch's new treatment for tuberculosis was premature, as we shall see later (Chapter 20). Patients were not cured, and many were made worse by the reactions that they experienced to the injected tuberculin. Koch, ever the observant scientist, recognized that these reactions might have diagnostic value. In his November 1890 paper, he reported, "the symptoms of reaction. . . . occurred without exception in all cases where a tuberculous process was present in the organism, . . . and I think I am justified in saying that the remedy will therefore in the future form an indispensable *aid* to diagnosis." If Koch was in error concerning the therapeutic efficacy of his tuberculin, he was dead on target with respect to its diagnostic use. With little change, it remains today the cornerstone of the familiar tuberculin ("TB") skin test. Within a year, Koch had completed further experiments with the alcohol solubility of tuberculin.[3] From the basis of today's knowledge, we recognize that Koch was the first to demonstrate that the immunologic activity of tuberculin resides primarily in its protein constituents.

The value of tuberculin as, in Koch's words, "an indispensable aid to diagnosis," was rapidly validated by the experience of doctors who observed that their patients developed fever when injected with Koch's tuberculin. However, this tuberculin reaction was first used for diagnosis in clinical practice not by physicians but by veterinarians who were concerned with widely prevalent bovine tuberculosis in cattle. Within a year of Koch's report German veterinarians were using tuberculin to diagnose tuberculous infection in animals.[4] Careful autopsies demonstrated that cattle reacting to tuberculin injected into the skin invariably proved to have lesions of tuberculosis, albeit often few and small. Transmission of bovine tuberculosis to humans was recognized as a threat to public health. Indeed, this subject was the source of considerable debate at the 1908 tuberculosis conference in Washington attended by Koch (Chapter 9), and within a decade the tuberculin skin testing of dairy herds had become widely practiced. Animals identified by this test as infected with tubercle bacilli were removed from herds and slaughtered. As early as 1896, the Massachusetts legislature appropriated money to compensate the owners of dairy herds whose animals were found to be tuberculin positive and killed, and the eradication campaign soon spread widely. The results were dramatic. In 1909, nineteen percent of seventeen hundred cattle in the District of Columbia were found to be infected.[5] By 1917 fewer than one percent of animals were infected, and in 1925 no animals reacted to tuberculin.

The Austrian physician, Clemens Freiherr Baron von Pirquet, was the first to use Koch's tuberculin in a skin test in humans. Born in 1874 in a small Austrian village, a landed aristocrat, and perhaps the most respected pediatrician of his day in Europe, von Pirquet is remembered as the father of the science and clinical specialty of allergy. Indeed, he invented the term allergy, first proposing its use in 1906.[6] Von Pirquet knew that individuals receiving Jenner's vaccination against small pox reacted differently at the inoculation site on the skin when they were revaccinated than they did upon first exposure to the vaccine. He reasoned that the skin of patients with tuberculosis might also react differently to tuberculin than did uninfected persons. And so he tried testing tuberculous children with tuberculin using a scratch or prick skin testing technique that he had developed to identify offending substances capable of evoking allergic reactions. In this fashion, he made the leap from a test that required injection of large amounts of tuberculin and the measurement of body temperature following the injection to a simple and easily read tuberculin skin test.

On May 8, 1907, von Pirquet reported to the Medical Society of Berlin that, "if a tuberculous child is inoculated . . . with tuberculin, a small papule occurs at the site of the inoculation that is light red at the beginning, gradually becomes dark red, and fades within eight days."[7] The following autumn, in a paper read before the Chicago Medical Society on October 14, 1908 and published three months later by the *Journal of the American Medical Association*, he described the results he had obtained by performing tuberculin skin tests on fourteen hundred and seven Viennese children.[8] He observed that essentially all children whom he considered "manifestly tuberculous" gave reactions to the tuberculin skin test. These reactions did not develop immediately, as he had already demonstrated to be the usual response in skin testing persons suffering from allergy with an offending substance. Rather, he noted delayed reactions when he examined the children on the two days following the test application. Today, we commonly refer to reactions taking one or two days to develop as delayed hypersensitivity, and we know that these reactions are a particular class of immunologic responses mediated by specific types of white blood cells.

Von Pirquet observed that many children who reacted to tuberculin were not apparently tuberculous. These children he considered to have latent or healed tuberculous lesions, which he concluded were "compatible with apparently perfect health." He adduced from his data that negative tuberculin skin tests generally meant an absence of prior tuberculous infection. For practical purposes, the tuberculin skin test as it is usually performed and interpreted today, had been born. It remained only for Mantoux, in the same year—1908, to substitute injection of the tuberculin material from a syringe for von Pirquet's needle scratch technique. "Tine tests," frequently used in doctors' offices today, are actually closer in technique to the one used by von Pirquet than the more precise Mantoux test.

In his landmark paper, von Pirquet made several other observations about tuberculin reactions and childhood tuberculosis that have withstood the test of time. He noted that almost all children infected before the age of two did not heal their infections but progressed to develop "manifest" tuberculosis. He noted that children with widely disseminated tuberculosis of a form that pathologists had come to call miliary[9] had negative tuberculin test reactions despite their extensive disease, and he noted that children with measles invariably had negative tuberculin reactions. He also reported that the frequency of positive tuberculin skin tests increased with the age of children tested, presumably because older children were more likely to have been exposed to and infected by tubercle bacilli. This observation led him to suggest that reactions in children could be used as an indicator of the amount of tuberculosis in the community. Finally, he concluded his presentation by proposing that healthy children should be tested in schools as a means of screening them for tuberculosis.

Von Pirquet's great contributions were recognized in his lifetime, and he received much public acclaim. His work was admired by the distinguished American academic medical leaders William Osler and William Welch[10] of Johns Hopkins University in Baltimore. They offered him a coveted professorship in pediatrics at Johns Hopkins University in 1909. He assumed this position with enthusiasm, but returned to Vienna after only a year. Later, he accepted a similar position at the University of Minnesota, again relinquishing it to return to Austria. Much of his apparent restlessness may have reflected his wife's unstable psychiatric state, and there is reason to suppose that he also may have had recurring bouts of depression. In 1929, Maria and Clemens von Pirquet died of cyanide poisoning in a double suicide.

By the time of von Pirquet's death, tuberculin skin testing had become widely accepted. In 1931, Florence Seibert, a biochemist working at the Henry Phipps Institute of the University of Pennsylvania,[11] began a series of studies designed to find "the active principal" of Koch's tuberculin. Her studies resulted in the preparation of a product from tuberculin named purified protein derivative, then and now commonly called PPD. While scarcely purified by modern chemical standards and while containing many substances other than protein, PPD has proven to be remarkably effective as a tuberculin skin test reagent. By 1934, Seibert had developed a standard method for the preparation of PPD. In 1941, she and John Glenn of the Mulford Laboratories of Sharp and Dohme prepared a single enormously large batch, half of which was set aside for research purposes, the other half of which was deposited with the United States Bureau of Standards and the World Health Organization. It serves to this day as the reference standard against which all other subsequent batches of PPD by all manufacturers are calibrated.

While Seibert's quest for "*the* active principal" of PPD was unsuccessful, she did identify three proteins and two polysaccharides in PPD having activity in skin tests. Research in this field has subsequently shown that there are many constituents of tuberculin, most of them proteins, that are active in eliciting tuberculin reactions.[12] That is, the reactivity that infected persons develop is not restricted to a single substance but is directed to many chemical components of tubercle bacilli. All such substances are termed "antigens" by immunologists.

As experience with tuberculin skin testing mounted, so also did problems associated with this diagnostic test. It soon became apparent that not everyone with a positive skin test was infected with tubercle bacilli and that not everyone infected with tubercle bacilli had a positive tuberculin test. False positive, "no lesion reactors" among slaughtered cattle threatened the continuation of programs to control bovine tuberculosis and prompted research studies that showed that animals inoculated with mycobacteria other than *Mycobacterium tuberculosis*, the tubercle bacillus, developed positive tuberculin tests. Epidemiologic studies among persons in North America showed that small positive reactions were especially common in the Southeastern United States and that these small reactions were similar to the those of no lesion reactor cattle.

To understand the cause of small false positive reactions, we have to recognize that the tuberculosis germ is one species—*Mycobacterium tuberculosis*—among many species of organisms belonging to the genus *Mycobacterium*. For a moment consider cats. There are many cats—lions, leopards, tigers, and alley cats. Some cats are vicious predators, some are domesticated pets. Similarly, some mycobacteria are vicious causes of disease and some are harmless. The harmless organisms are widespread, many residing in soil and water, and all people meet harmless mycobacteria every day. All mycobacteria share some antigens—substances that elicit delayed skin test reactions. Within the array of antigens possessed by an individual species of mycobacteria, some are quite specific, but some are shared widely. Thus, it is not surprising that some or many persons, perhaps most persons, develop delayed hypersensitivity to some of the antigens of mycobacteria other than the tubercle bacillus. For the most part, the tuberculin skin test has been calibrated by adjusting the dose of PPD given so that these weak nonspecific cross-reactions are not recognized. However, in some parts of the world, including most of the coastal areas of the southeastern United States, it is not possible to avoid these nonspecifically positive tests, and in these geographic regions tuberculin testing has limited value for the diagnosis of tuberculous infection.

Most middle aged American readers of this book will recall having been tuberculin skin tested in school; younger readers will not. As the prevalence of tuberculous infection has declined to low levels in the United States, the prevalence of nonspecific tuberculin reactivity has remained unchanged. Thus, in recent years, positive tuberculin reactions in otherwise healthy individuals not exposed to persons with tuberculosis have become more frequently a manifestation of nonspecific delayed hypersensitivity to some other mycobacterium than one of tuberculous infection. The decline of tuberculosis has made this potent screening test developed by von Pirquet and others less and less predictive of tuberculous infection. Routine testing of children in schools, first suggested by von Pirquet and later widely practiced in the United States, has now disappeared.

The other problem with tuberculin tests—negative reactions in persons who obviously had been infected—was also geographically defined. In the Ohio and Mississippi River valleys large numbers of persons were identified who had obvious healed and calcified foci of tuberculosis visible in their chest radiographs but who did not react to tuberculin. Nursing students were being carefully screened, for their risk of developing tuberculosis was especially great, and it was difficult to understand how so many of these young persons with scars in their lungs failed to react to tuberculin. Not until the mid 1950s was it recognized that asymptomatic infections with *Histoplasma capsulatum*, a generally harmless soil fungus common in the drainage area of the Ohio and Mississippi rivers, healed to produce scars that radiologists could not distinguish from healed tuberculosis. In Cincinnati it was found that eight out of ten young adults had been infected with *Histoplasma*. In the Sonoran desert areas of California and neighboring southwestern states, the soil fungus *Coccidioides imitus* took the place of midwestern *H. capsulatum*. Abnormal chest radiographs due to these clinically unimportant infections were common, and they were being confused with tuberculosis. When this situation was recognized, the tuberculin skin test was vindicated.

In 1958 the United States Public Health Service and the United States Navy began testing all American naval recruits as they entered the service. Continued over many years, this program allowed Lydia Edwards and her colleagues to establish a county-by-county atlas of tuberculin skin test reactivity in the United States.[13] This atlas provided an accurate picture of the geographic distribution of tuberculous infection in the United States, and it provided data to permit rational targeting of disease control programs.

As we attempt to understand tuberculosis, the most important lesson to be learned from the story of the tuberculin skin test is that there is a difference between being infected with tubercle bacilli and being sick from this infection. As von Pirquet recognized, many individuals are harmlessly infected. These persons are not sick and are not contagious to others. They do not have disease. In the world, they are many. In fact, one-third of the global population is so infected. In technologically advanced North America and Europe, they are relatively few.

It is important to note that of all of those infected with the germ that causes tuberculosis, only about one in twelve to one in twenty will ever develop the disease caused by this bacterium. Some of those who do will meet their fate at an early age, as did Maria Brontë. Some will harbor their silent infections for decades, as did Eleanor Roosevelt, before succumbing. Interestingly, for those persons like Eleanor Roosevelt who have sustained an early primary infection, the threat is usually not from another infection, for the primary infection brings with it a degree of protective immunity. Although they may walk in the valley of the shadow of death, they fear no evil. Rather, they are constantly threatened by the shadow that goes in and out with them, a break-down of their healed primary lesion and the development of reactivation tuberculosis. It is the interplay between this host immunity and the tubercle bacillus that becomes the captain of the fate of infected persons. The fact that the majority of infected individuals who enter the ring of combat with tuberculosis are victors in the struggle is of great importance to our understanding of this disease. It is also important not to forget that the battle is not one defined by a set number of rounds. An entire lifetime may pass before the final bell and before it is known whether the tubercle bacillus or the immune host is to be victorious.

14

A Family Affair

When Chopin was ostracized on Mallorca, Georges Sand was surprised that the Spanish islanders considered tuberculosis to be an infectious disease. In northern Europe the prevailing view was that tuberculosis was an hereditary condition. In fact, this view had been accepted for centuries by most people, and the contrary view that it was caused by an infectious agent was not seriously entertained by most medical authorities until Koch's studies made any other idea untenable. How else but by invoking heredity could one explain the remarkable spread of tuberculosis through the Brontë family that we have noted in Chapter 4? Not knowing of the long and variable incubation period of tuberculosis, one could not expect an infectious disease spread by contact to crop up at such different times and ages in the six Brontë children.

Koch's ideas and experiments inexorably pushed aside all other theories of the cause of consumption. Tuberculosis is an infectious disease caused by a well defined germ that bears the scientific name *Mycobacterium tuberculosis* and is known to all as the tubercle bacillus. In some parts of the world, it is still known as "Koch's bacillus." This does not, however, mean that inborn, genetically determined factors do not influence this disease and its human manifestations. Consider Keats and Stevenson. Surely something in their genetic make-ups set the courses their illnesses sailed. Both poets had family histories of tuberculosis. Both may have been infected by their mothers. Keats succumbed rapidly from a background of vigorous health. Stevenson lived for years with chronic illness. It is hard not to believe that the individual constitutions—the inherited genetic make-ups—of these two men did not determine their fates. Modern science supports this view, and the studies of Max Lurie provided the initial underpinnings for this support.

Max Bernard Lurie was born in Telshee, Lithuania on September 12,

1893, the son of a rabbi. His family traced its origins to Talmudic scholars of the eleventh century. In 1907, the Lurie family emigrated to the
United States, settling first in Lowell, Massachusetts and later in New York
City. Lurie became a naturalized American citizen in 1914. He attended
the College of the City of New York and received the Bachelor of Arts
degree in 1917. Eschewing the family rabbinical tradition, he entered
medical school at Cornell University, earning the M.D. degree in 1921.[1]

Lurie's mother died of tuberculosis. Before her, her father and her
grandmother had succumbed to this disease. What then must the young
Max Lurie have thought when he developed tuberculosis as a senior
medical student? Whatever he thought, he knew what he must do. In
his words, "I diagnosed it and took myself out to Colorado. But I tried
to get well there and be a full-time intern at the same time. The outcome was I became a patient at the National Jewish Hospital in Denver."[2]

Lurie spent the next five years engaged in research on tuberculosis at
the National Jewish Hospital, and in 1926 he joined the Department
of Pathology of the Phipps Institute at the University of Pennsylvania in
Philadelphia.[3] There he undertook a series of studies that spanned four
decades and provided the basis for much of our understanding of the
influences of genes upon the development of tuberculosis. The importance of his work was recognized in 1953 when the University of
Montreal awarded him the Claude Bernard Medal and again in 1956
when the National Tuberculosis Association presented him with its coveted Trudeau Medal. Max Lurie was still engaged in his studies when he
died of heart failure in 1966 at the age of seventy-three.

Mindful of his own family history, Lurie was convinced that heredity
played a major role in the development of tuberculosis. He chose to
study this subject in families of rabbits.[4] Why rabbits? The aptness of
this species was suggested to him by his mentor at the Phipps Institute,
Eugene L. Opie. Lurie was intrigued that "the rabbit's marked resistance to the human bacillus and its very great susceptibility to the bovine organism presented the possibility of shedding some light not only
on organ resistance but also on species resistance. Furthermore, since
the rabbit shares with man many of the characteristic responses to the
infection, the host-parasite relationships revealed in this animal might
have some significance for the understanding of the nature of human
disease."[5] Today, one might well argue that there are better animals than
rabbits in which to study the lymphocyte-mediated immunology so

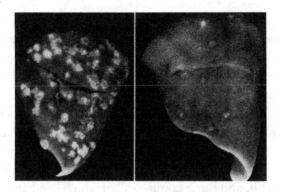

Figure 14.1. Left lungs removed from susceptible (left) and resistant (right) rabbits by Dr. Max Lurie four weeks after the inhalation of large numbers of human tubercle bacilli. Although the resistant rabbit actually inhaled twenty-four percent more bacilli than the susceptible rabbit, it developed many fewer tubercles, as is evident in the photographs showing the surfaces of the lungs. Careful study revealed that the two lungs of the susceptible rabbit contained seven times as many tubercles as the two lungs of the resistant rabbit. Lurie MB, Zappasodi R, Tickner C. On the nature of genetic resistance to tuberculosis in the light of the host-parasite relationships in natively resistent and susceptible rabbits. Am Rev Tuberc Pulm Dis 1955; 72:297–329. Figure reproduced with the permission of the American Lung Association.

important in the development of tuberculosis, but it is true that bovine tuberculosis in rabbits is more akin to human disease in its chronic course than any other animal form of tuberculosis.

From the research laboratories of several colleagues, Lurie obtained rabbits with pedigrees known for five or more generations. He bred these rabbits to develop families that he carefully studied over many subsequent generations. None of these rabbit families were related, and all had a substantial degree of in-breeding. Lurie found that the members of some of these families were highly susceptible to tuberculosis when infected with bovine tubercle bacilli; other families were relatively resistant. As he continued to in-breed these families, their susceptibility and resistance profiles did not change in succeeding generations. Lurie conducted many insightful and revealing studies of the pathogenesis of tuberculosis in his rabbits. Standing most prominently among his observations was one salient point. Some of Lurie's rabbit families, like the Keats and Brontë families, carried an obvious genetic predisposition to tuberculosis. Others, emulating Stevenson, carried an equally obvious genetic resistance to tuberculosis. Related rabbits bred to carry similar genes displayed similar resistance or susceptibility to tuberculosis.

Mice are easier to breed through many generations than rabbits, and mice also come in strains with differing susceptibilities to tuberculosis. Emil Skamene and his colleagues in Montreal studied the susceptibility of mice to BCG, a vaccine strain of the bovine tubercle bacillus (Chapter 15), and found it to be chiefly related to a single gene.[6] Indeed, they were able to isolate this gene and determine its DNA composition.[7]

Setting aside rabbits and mice and setting aside the remarkable Brontë, Keats, Stevenson, and Lurie families, all of which lived and experienced tuberculosis in times when exposure was extraordinarily common, can we find evidence in human history to support the idea that some people—perhaps most people who become sick with tuberculosis—carry a genetic predisposition to this disease? Scientific investigators have approached this question in a number of ways, but the most direct answers come from studies of twins. There have been several such studies, and the conclusions have generally been similar. Let us examine one conducted in England in 1952 and carefully reanalyzed twenty-five years later using more modern statistical methods by George Comstock, the dean of American epidemiologists interested in tuberculosis.[8]

Twins come in two varieties. Identical twins—monozygotic in scientific terminology—are the result of a fertilized egg that splits into two halves, each half going on to produce a normal embryo. These twins share all of the same genes, for they started as one. They are always of the same sex, the same blood groups, and in every way are so much the product of their genetic sameness that even their parents may find it hard to tell them apart. They would be expected to have the same propensity for tuberculosis, if susceptibility to tuberculosis were influenced by heredity. Nonidentical or fraternal twins—dizygotic to biologists—are the result of the fertilization of two separate eggs, each of which goes on to produce a healthy fetus and infant. They are related to each other in the same way that all brothers and sisters are related and no more alike than any other two siblings with the same parents. They might share some familial disposition to disease, but not to the same degree that identical twins would. If reared in the same home by the same parents, both types of twins might share predisposing environmental factors, but only identical twins could share genetic factors.

Studies conducted in the first half of the twentieth century had compared identical and fraternal twins with respect to tuberculosis and concluded that there were genetic factors important in determining susceptibility to tuberculosis. Feeling that there were serious errors in the methods used for analysis of these original studies, the Royal College of Physicians of London commissioned Dr. Barbara Simonds to conduct another study; because of her illness and death, the study was completed by her husband. The results were published in 1963. The study concluded that if one twin had tuberculosis, then tuberculosis was more likely to develop in an identical than a fraternal twin sibling. However, the Simonds' analysis concluded that this result probably resulted from closer contact of identical than fraternal twins, not from genetic relatedness. This study and the Simonds' conclusions stood alone in opposition to the prevailing view that genes influenced susceptibility to tuberculosis.

George Comstock noted that computers were not available to the Simonds as they tabulated and analyzed data from nearly twenty-two thousand questionnaires sent to tuberculosis patients and the histories of more than four hundred pairs of twins. Moreover, the introduction of computers had permitted the development and application of newer and more sophisticated methods of statistical analysis. And so he undertook to reanalyze the Simonds' data on two hundred and two twin pairs that remained after careful and critical review of the original survey data.[9] Tuberculosis occurred slightly more than twice as frequently in the identical twin sibling of a patient with tuberculosis than it did in the nonidentical twin sibling of such a patient. Adjustment for a variety of factors that might have influenced the results failed to change the outcome. Genes were back in their place as major determinants of susceptibility to tuberculosis. Whether rabbit, mouse, or human, your family history is important in determining what happens to you if you become infected with the tubercle bacillus.

If the genes in your family tree are important to your battle with the tubercle bacillus, what of the genes associated with your race? It certainly seems a reasonable question to ask. The answer is not so easily obtained, however, because it is not easy to separate environmental circumstances from genetic susceptibility when comparing tuberculosis in different racial groups. I believe that it is best to approach this challenging topic by dividing the problem into three questions: Does your race influence the likelihood of becoming infected if you are exposed to tubercle bacilli? Does your race influence the likelihood of developing disease if you are infected? And does your race influence the course of your illness if you develop disease? At least for people of African and Caucasian descent—and I will focus primarily on this major racial difference because there are more data relevant to it available than there are for other racial differences—the answers to the three questions appear to me to be probably not, possibly so, and probably yes.

William Stead is one of the great contemporary observers of the natural history of tuberculosis. From his vantage point in the Arkansas Department of Health, he has observed tuberculosis as it has occurred in nursing homes in Arkansas. He and his coworkers noted that among more than thirteen thousand persons admitted to two hundred and twenty-seven nursing homes in Arkansas, conversion of the tuberculin skin test from negative to positive, a marker for infection with tuberculosis germs, occurred nearly twice as often in African Americans as in white Americans.[10] After an extensive analysis, they concluded that this difference could only be explained if African Americans were more susceptible to infection than white Americans when exposed to tubercle bacilli in the air.

In 1990 an outbreak of tuberculosis occurred in an elementary school in Missouri in which exposure of children of the two races was almost certainly equal.[11] A physical education teacher developed tuberculosis that was unrecognized for most of an entire school year. Of more than three hundred children in the school, half had positive tuberculin skin tests, and thirty-two children had abnormal chest radiographs indicating tuberculosis. The infection rates in white and African American children were equal. Frequency of exposure to the diseased teacher was an important determinant of infection; race was not.

Stead's study in nursing homes makes many unstated assumptions about the similarity of exposure to tuberculosis in nursing homes of African Americans and white Americans. So also, but to a lesser extent, did the study of Missouri school children. On balance, the results from the school study seem more credible to me, and I conclude that race has little or no effect on susceptibility to tuberculous infection when conditions of exposure are the same.

Now let us recall that the vast majority of individuals infected with tubercle bacilli remain healthy and let us look at the risk of disease in infected persons of different races. If populations of different races could be studied in the same environment, then one might be able to sort out the relative importance of heredity and living circumstances on the development of tuberculosis. Julius Katz and Solomon Kunofsky of the New York State Health Department recognized that nonsegregated state mental hospitals might provide an opportunity for a study of this type, and in 1960 they published a report of investigations they carried out in patients from New York City who were hospitalized in state mental hospitals and subsequently developed tuberculosis.[12] During the decade before they began their study, tuberculosis case rates for African Americans in New York City were four times those for white Americans. When hospitalized in the same mental hospital wards, tuberculosis rates in these people fell, and those in African Americans fell dramatically so that they were only about fifty percent greater than those in white Americans. With further time, this difference declined to about thirty percent. The interpretation of this study was quite clear. Environmental circumstances had much more to do with the risk of infected persons developing tuberculosis than did race. Before we close the book on this subject, however, we must also deal with the fact that large racial differences have persisted in the American population through a time period in history when environmental differences have been narrowing.

The laboratory studies of Alfred Crowle may have a bearing on this issue. The primary defense cell of the body responsible for forming granulomas and for containing the growth and spread of tubercle bacilli from the site of original infection to areas of disease is the macrophage. Circulating in the blood as monocytes, these cells are called into infected tissues by lymphocytes where they change into macrophages and attack foreign invaders, including tubercle bacilli. Crowle, using imaginative and elegant techniques with their roots in the hanging drop cultures of Koch, studied the replication of tubercle bacilli within human macrophages from the blood of African American and white persons.[13] When initially introduced, tubercle bacilli were more rapidly killed by macrophages from African Americans than from white Americans. However, once growing within cells, the germs grew more rapidly in monocytes and macrophages from African American than white American persons. If these laboratory results can be applied to living beings—

always an assumption one must make with care—then they suggest that tubercle bacilli might grow more rapidly and have a better chance of escaping the containing action of macrophages in persons of African descent than those of Caucasian descent and hence be more likely to cause disease.

Finally, what of the form and progression of tuberculosis as related to race? Arnold Rich was one of America's greatest pathologists and students of tuberculosis. His book on this disease was a pace-setting accomplishment that heralded the application of modern scientific inquiry into the mechanisms of this disease.[14] In his text he carefully documents a tendency for people of African descent to have more florid lymph node enlargement with tuberculosis than do similarly diseased people of Caucasian origin. This observation has been verified by others, and this difference must mean some racially-connected, genetic difference in how the body handles tubercle bacilli.

Throughout this book I have tried to relate history to modern concepts of the pathogenesis of tuberculosis. History may have something further to teach us about susceptibility to tuberculosis, and it is useful to return to history in trying to sort out the impact of genetics upon the epidemic spread of tuberculosis among naive populations. The challenge is to decide why tuberculosis spreads so dramatically following its introduction into populations that have not seen this disease in hundreds of years. Is it simply a matter of how many previously uninfected, susceptible individuals there are in a population waiting to become infected at the time of the introduction of an infectious disease? Or is it because a high prevalence of tuberculosis over many generations leads to the evolution of an entire race of people that is genetically resistant and that without this natural selection a people evolves that is unusually susceptible? Stated otherwise, is it a matter of genes selected by evolution or lymphocytes sensitized by exposure?

Some of the most relevant historical evidence on tuberculosis and populations comes from reports of early contact between Europeans, whose continent was awash with tuberculosis, and other peoples to whom the disease was essentially unknown.[15] We have seen, in Chapter 4, that tuberculosis devastated the residents of Pitcairn Island when it was introduced there. S. Lyle Cummins, a Professor of Pathology at the Royal Army Medical College of London, reviewed the evidence for tuberculosis in many isolated societies.[16] He gives examples of places that were described as essentially free of the disease by early writers, only to have the disease spread rapidly upon its introduction in a manner to suggest that the particular ethnic group must have been unusually susceptible to tuberculosis. Some of his accounts are more credible than others.

Cummins states that tuberculosis was "quite unknown" in the steppes of Russia in 1886. Yet he presents data demonstrating that more than forty percent of women and sixty percent of men were infected with tubercle bacilli in these isolated regions twenty-five years later. In fact, since age specific infection rates are given, it is possible to estimate the annual risk of infection among these Tartar people at the beginning of the twentieth century. It was about eight percent per year, a high figure that would indicate new cases developing at a rate of three to four hundred per one hundred thousand persons per year. Today, such high case rates are seen in parts of Africa, the Philippines, Haiti, the Andean altiplano, and a only a few other places.

We can view Cummins' report in two ways. We can suppose that the early assumption that tuberculosis was rare among the people of the Russian steppes was incorrect, noting that it is based on what can hardly have been more than casual observations. Alternatively, we can conclude that a tuberculosis epidemic spread among these people with lightning speed. Such a firestorm of epidemic tuberculosis did occur among the indigenous peoples of the Arctic after the disease was introduced to them. Neither on the Russian steppes nor the Arctic tundra does one need to invoke genetic or racial factors, yet in each they might well have contributed.

Borrel, in an often quoted paper,[17] wrote of tuberculosis among black troops from Senegal enrolled in the French army during the first world war. In the camps in France where these African men were living in barracks and receiving military training, thirteen hundred and fifteen deaths due to tuberculosis occurred in 1916 through 1919. Borrel tells us that there were approximately fifty thousand Senegalese soldiers housed at these camps. Of course, the relevant question is how much tuberculosis was present in Senegal at the time. That is, did these soldiers come to France as uninfected persons who then succumbed to a disease introduced into their naive bodies by their French comrades in arms? Or were they already infected and did they then undergo a high break-down rate because of the crowded living conditions in their bar-racks? And in either case, were racial or other genetic characteristics of the Senegalese men important? Borrel cites observations made in 1912 by Calmette, an eminent French physician and scientist whom we will meet in the next chapter. Calmette found that four to seven percent of rural Senegalese reacted in Von Pirquet's tuberculin test. This low figure was cited by Borrel and Cummings to characterize the Senegalese sol-diers as a naive, previously unexperienced population with respect to tuberculosis. However, Calmette also found that twenty to thirty per-cent of urban Senegalese gave positive reactions, a high figure bespeak-ing substantial prior contact with tubercle bacilli. We do not know where the conscripts who developed tuberculosis came from. The Senegalese population was a mixed one, then, and we must be cautions in drawing conclusions from it.

Whether or not race is an important factor, it is hard to escape the repeated observations that tuberculosis has a propensity to sweep through naive populations at an alarming rate, whether in the Arctic, the steppes of Russia, or Pitcairn Island. One can look to more than one possible explanation to understand the rapid spread. It might be that a large number of uninfected and hence nonimmune persons in the popula-tion present an easy target for the tubercle bacillus. Or it might be that Darwinian natural selection produces a more resistant population when tubercle bacilli are constantly present. Some authorities accept this lat-ter hypothesis; others challenge it on the basis of what is known of the distribution of tuberculosis in early times, the number of generations that must have passed for resistant strains of humans to have evolved, and the failure of people to develop resistance in countries such as Haiti where tuberculosis has probably been present for hundreds of years with case rates remaining very high to the present.[18]

What can we conclude from Lurie's rabbits, from twins, from epi-demics in naive peoples, and from outbreaks in children? The inherited traits of an individual—genes—are important. To misquote Hamlet,[19] there are genes that shape our ends, rough-hew them how we will. Genes determine the risk of disease and its course; I believe that they do not influence the risk of infection when an individual is exposed. These genes relate to family, probably to race, and possibly to the prior experi-ence of a people with this disease.

15

Bacille Calmette Guérin

Immunization is by far the most effective disease prevention measure. Millions of children are protected by their baby shots, and mass immunization campaigns have eradicated small pox from the world and polio from the western hemisphere. A global polio eradication campaign based on vaccination is under way, and measles is the next target. Why not tuberculosis?

The story begins two centuries ago. When Mary Wortly Montagu, the wife of the British Ambassador to Turkey, travelled to Asia Minor, she learned that a practice termed variolation (variola is the Latin name for small pox) was in wide-spread use for the prevention of small pox. The practice was to introduce a small amount of pustular or scabrous material from the skin lesions of patients with small pox into the skin of the arm or some other preferred site of persons who had never had the disease by scratching with a needle. The inoculated persons then developed a mild case of small pox on the eighth day and had a limited illness lasting two to three days. Thereafter, they were immune to further attacks of this disease, however often they might be exposed. When Lady Montagu returned to her home country, she brought news of this medical practice, and it soon became widely used in Europe. No one could doubt that immunity from the dread small pox was worth the cost of two or three sick days.[1]

William Jenner, a noted and respected English physician, knew of variolation. He also knew that milk maids who had suffered from cow pox did not develop small pox when exposed. Cow pox was a skin disease of the udders of dairy cattle, and those who milked these cattle developed lesions on their hands and a mild illness of one to four days. Jenner decided to see if this infection did, indeed, protect against small pox. On May 14, 1796, in his words, he "selected a healthy boy, about eight years old, for the purpose of inoculating for the cow-pox." He inserted pus from the lesions of a dairy maid into two superficial cuts which he made on the arms of this boy. Jenner then reported, "On the seventh day he complained of uneasiness . . . and the ninth he became a little chilly, lost his appetite, and had a slight headache. . . . on the day following, he was perfectly well." On July 1, Jenner inoculated the boy with virulent small pox pustular material. He did so again several months later. No disease resulted from these inoculations of small pox. The boy was immune, and vaccination, essentially as we know it today, was born.[2]

The term vaccination derives from vaccinia, the Latin name for cow pox. We now use the word in a general sense for all immunizations designed to prevent disease. Louis Pasteur suggested this usage as an honor to Jenner's first immunization of a human.

Late in the nineteenth century, Pasteur, an already famous French microbiologist, became interested in rabies. He attempted to attenuate the rabies virus—to render it less virulent—by passing it through rabbits. He took ground up infected spinal cord from rabid dogs and injected it into rabbits. As these rabbits became diseased, he injected material from them into other rabbits. When he finally reinjected it back into dogs after passage through a series of rabbits, it no longer produced rabies in the dogs. Moreover, the animals were immune to rabies. Pasteur had developed a crude vaccine against rabies.

By 1885, Pasteur had immunized fifty dogs without untoward event. He was then sixty-three years old and famous, but he was in ill health and handicapped by the residuals of a stroke he had suffered some years earlier. On July 6 of that year a family presented at his door, bringing to him a nine year old boy named Joseph Meister who had been badly bitten on the legs and hands by a rabid dog two days before. The boy had fourteen separate wounds, and some on the legs were so deep that he could not walk. A local surgeon had attempted to sterilize the wounds by pouring carbolic acid on them. On that memorable day, Pasteur attended the regular meeting of the Académie de Sciences. He told two of his colleagues about his young patient, and they returned with Pasteur and examined the child. All agreed the boy was doomed to die of rabies.

Pasteur was ready to act. At 8 PM on July 6, sixty hours after the boy had been bitten, Pasteur injected his attenuated rabbit rabies virus into the boy. He gave the lad twelve additional inoculations over the subsequent ten days. Joseph Meister remained well. He was immune to rabies, an invariably fatal disease for which there was then and still is no treatment. So convinced was Pasteur that he had successfully immunized his young patient, that he later inoculated the boy with virulent canine rabies, from which the youngster suffered no illness. "Since the middle of August," Pasteur wrote in his account of these events, "I have looked forward with confidence to the future good health of Joseph Meister. At the present time, three months and three weeks have elapsed since the accident, his state of health leaves nothing to be desired. . . ."[3]

Knowing of the earlier work of Jenner and Pasteur, Robert Koch was understandably eager to develop a vaccine for tuberculosis. He did his studies in guinea pigs. The type of immune reaction he observed has become known as the Koch phenomenon. As he described it:

"If a healthy guinea pig is inoculated with a pure culture of tubercle bacilli, the inoculation wound usually closes and appears to heal within a few days; however, after ten to fourteen days a hard nodule appears and soon breaks down to form an ulcer which remains until the animal dies. By contrast, something quite different happens when a guinea pig already ill with tuberculosis is inoculated. . . . In such an animal the small inoculation wound also closes initially but no nodule develops; instead, a peculiar change occurs at the inoculation site over the next day or two. . . . During the following few days the altered skin becomes necrotic and sloughs off, leaving a flat ulcer which usually heals rapidly and permanently without involvement of the neighboring lymph nodes. Hence, the inoculated tubercle bacilli affect the skin of a healthy animal in a quite different manner than that of a tuberculous one."[4]

These guinea pig studies underlay Koch's claims of therapeutic efficacy for tuberculin (Chapter 20) and his dream of a cure for that disease.

Thus, the twentieth century dawned with the concepts of immunity and vaccination to induce immunity firmly in their scientific place. Koch's experiments made it clear that immunity existed to tuberculosis as well as to other infectious diseases. The time was ripe for the development of a vaccine against tuberculosis, and the task was undertaken by Albert Calmette and Camille Guérin.

By any measure and even in the remarkable half century of Koch and

Pasteur that gave birth to the science of microbiology, Léon Charles Albert Calmette was a remarkable man. Born in Nice on July 12, 1863, he was educated as a naval medical officer and served in the Far East, where he carried out studies of the parasitic disease filariasis that earned him early attention. After his return to France and marriage to Émilie de la Salle, he continued his studies at the Pasteur Institute in Paris. On the recommendation of Pasteur himself, Calmette was assigned to direct a recently opened Pasteur Institute in Saigon. There he distinguished himself in conducting a small pox vaccination campaign and in studies of snake venoms. When the French government opened a new Pasteur Institute for medical research at Lille near the Belgian border in 1895, Calmette, who had recently returned to France, accepted the call to become its Director.[5]

Calmette recognized that tuberculosis was a major health problem of the industrial city of Lille, and he determined to work on this disease in his new institute. He was joined in this work by Camille Guérin. Jean Marie Camille Guérin was born in Poitiers on December 22, 1872. Influenced by his step-father, he trained in veterinary medicine at the École Alfort near Paris, a veterinary school directed by the noted microbiologist Edmond Nocard. He finished his training in 1896, and with Nocard's sponsorship he obtained a post as Calmette's research assistant.[6]

Calmette and Guérin began their work on tuberculosis about 1900. The development of a vaccine was their clearly perceived goal. They observed serendipitously that adding ox bile to the liquid medium in which they were cultivating tubercle bacilli lowered its virulence, and this gave them the hope that they might produce a strain of tubercle bacilli of low virulence—attenuated, in the terminology of vaccine makers. Such an attenuated strain might serve as the cow pox for tuberculosis.[7]

The two pioneering microbiologists chose to begin their vaccine production attempts with a strain of bovine tubercle bacilli that had originally been isolated from the udder of a tuberculous cow in 1902 by Guérin's mentor, Edmond Nocard. They cultured this strain on ox bile-containing medium, and after thirty-nine passages they noted a change in the appearance of the organism. The colonies were smoother and smaller. They began inoculating animals—guinea pigs, rabbits—and they became convinced that they had achieved a strain of tubercle bacilli of low virulence. By 1913, after eleven years of patient work, they were ready to vaccinate cows, the animals in which the ancestors of their vaccine strain had produced disease.

In 1914 war exploded across Europe, and Kaiser Wilhelm's armies soon overran northern France. Lille fell after a siege of ten days during which the city was shelled at a rate of one thousand rounds a day—an artillery shell every minute and one-half. Ironically, a nephew of Robert Koch, who had worked in Calmette's laboratory before the war, was among the officers leading the German troops.

The occupying Germans did not permit Calmette and Guérin to leave Lille, and the two men quietly continued their work on a tuberculosis vaccine. They inoculated nine cows with their vaccine and then infected them with virulent bovine tubercle bacilli. Before they could complete their experiments, however, the Germans requisitioned all cattle in Lille. With the collusion of German army veterinarians, Calmette and Guérin were able to kill and autopsy their nine animals. The results were striking. None of the animals had tuberculosis. Working secretly, beset by shortages of materials needed to make culture medium, but undaunted, Calmette and Guérin continued to culture and maintain their vaccine strain. By 1919 when the war ended, they had recultured their vaccine strain every three weeks through two hundred and thirty cultures and had tested it in guinea pigs, rabbits, cows, and horses.

The war brought personal tragedy to the two scientists. Guérin arranged for his children to be evacuated from war-torn northern France. His wife stayed with him, but she died before the end of the war. In 1917, the Germans began seizing French civilians as hostages to guarantee the safety of German prisoners of war held by the French. Émilie Calmette was among those taken, and she remained interned in Germany until after the armistice in 1919. Small wonder that Calmette became an embittered man in his later years, unwilling even to speak to German scientists. Calmette died in 1933, preoccupied at that time about the rising prominence of a German demagogue named Adolph Hitler.

With the return of peace to France, Calmette and Guérin resumed their studies of their attenuated strain of bovine tubercle bacilli. They found it to be safe in monkeys and chimpanzees. They named their bacterium *Bacilli Bilié Calmette-Guérin*; the word bilié was later dropped, and it became known as BCG, the name it carries to this day. The two scientists were convinced that their new vaccine was safe, and they believed it would be effective. They were ready to try it in humans, but they approached this step cautiously.

In 1921 Calmette and Guérin contacted Drs. Benjamin Weill-Hallé and Raymond Turpin at the Hôpital Charité in Paris to consider who might be an appropriate subject. Surely it must be an uninfected person who was, none-the-less, at extremely high risk of dying of tuberculosis, at a risk so high that one could make this first use of BCG in good conscience. For this first test they chose a newborn infant whose mother had died of tuberculosis a few hours after the baby's birth. The orphan child was to be raised by its grandmother, who also had advanced tuberculosis. Calmette and his colleagues at the Hôpital Charité knew that in this circumstance the baby would almost certainly become infected with tuberculosis and would very likely develop one of the fatal disseminated forms of this disease to which newborns are particularly susceptible. Thus, on July 18, 1921, they administered the first vaccine dose to this baby, feeding a culture of BCG to the three day old infant. They gave an additional doses on the fifth and seventh days of life. The child showed no ill effects and was raised in good health by its tuberculous grandmother.[8]

During the next few years, additional doses of BCG were given. By 1924, more than six hundred children had been vaccinated, and the Pasteur Institute in Lille began producing the vaccine in large amounts; by 1931 a special laboratory for BCG production had been established, with Guérin in charge. From 1924 to 1928, more than one hundred thousand doses were given to infants, all without serious complications. Calmette vaccinated his own ten grandchildren. The League of Nations certified BCG as safe for human use in 1928. In 1929 Calmette reported that the death rate of unvaccinated children of tuberculous parents was thirty-three percent while the rate for similarly exposed BCG-vaccinated children was less than four percent.[9] Albeit with caution, Calmette's results and BCG itself gained increasing acceptance. Throughout Europe and in Canada, committees were established to evaluate the new vaccine, and BCG came into increasing use; doctors in the United States were slower to accept it.[10]

Then disaster struck. The German City of Lübeck was engulfed in a major outbreak of tuberculosis. The Lübeck Health Department obtained a culture of BCG from the Pasteur Institute in Paris and began to prepare vaccine for use in that city. In March and April of 1930 this BCG prepared in Lübeck was given to two hundred and fifty-one young children. It soon became apparent that something was wrong. By October, seventy-two of the vaccinated children had died, all but five from tuberculosis. Calmette himself investigated this "catastrophe of Lübeck." He was able to obtain information on all but two of the vaccinated children. In addition to the sixty-seven children who had died of tuberculosis and the five who had died of other causes, one hundred and eight children were ill, many of them with probable tuberculosis. Only seventy-two remained healthy.[11]

What happened? Autopsies demonstrated that the bacteria that produced tuberculosis in these children were not BCG but were virulent human tubercle bacilli. Cultures found in the hospital laboratory where the vaccine doses were prepared contained not BCG but disease-producing tubercle bacilli. These virulent cultures were identified as a strain of human tubercle bacilli sent to Kiel from the Koch Institute in Berlin and then passed on to the Lübeck laboratory. The virulent strain had been kept in the same incubator as the cultures of BCG, and was inadequately labelled. The children of Lübeck had not been vaccinated. They had been given virulent tubercle bacilli, the result of a tragic mix-up in the hospital laboratory in Lübeck. Both French and German commissions investigating the tragedy exonerated BCG, but the reputation of the vaccine had been sorely damaged.

Despite the Lübeck catastrophe, BCG came into increasing use in Europe and elsewhere. It was clearly a safe vaccine. A number of small studies of its efficacy were carried out, but none meeting rigorous scientific standards until Dr. Joseph Aronson of the Phipps Institute[12] at the University of Pennsylvania addressed the problem.

The United States Public Health Service was and still is responsible for providing health care to indigenous native American Indians living on reservations. Tuberculosis case rates were high among these people, and their accessibility through the Public Health Service clinics made them a good population for study. Over a three year period from 1935 to 1938, Aronson and his colleagues tuberculin skin tested more than eight thousand of these individuals. Ninety percent of those in the twenty to twenty-four year old age group reacted to tuberculin, bespeaking an exceptionally high rate of infection with tubercle bacilli. Aronson then randomly divided the approximately three thousand nonreactors nineteen years old or younger into two groups, one group receiving BCG and the other a saline solution placebo. The Public Health Service then reexamined these trial participants every year for the next decade, repeating their tuberculin skin tests, examining them clinically, and obtaining radiographic examinations of their lungs. Subsequently, follow-up studies were conducted at five year intervals until twenty years of data had been gathered. More than ninety-nine percent of the participants were followed for the entire twenty year study period. Tuberculosis occurred in sixty-eight of the control subjects but in only thirteen of the BCG-vaccinated subjects. There could be little doubt that BCG was protective.[13]

World War II engulfed the entire globe, and the attention of medical and public health experts was focused on more urgent problems than that of tuberculosis. However, with the end of the war, attention turned back to tuberculosis, and for good reason. Tuberculosis epidemics have always flourished in the wake of war, and the immediate post-war years of the 1940s were no exception. Those years saw the rapid spread of this still dread disease in Europe. Poland was reeling in the wake of the armies that had marched across it and occupied it, and tuberculosis loomed as an urgent problem. The Poles turned to Denmark for help, and in January 1947 the Danish Red Cross began delivering BCG to the children of Poland. Led by Johannes Holm and working out of rudimentary facilities and under difficult logistic conditions, the Danes tuberculin tested more than two hundred thousand children, and gave BCG to forty-seven thousand uninfected youngsters.[14]

Johannes Holm was Chief of the Tuberculosis Division of the State Serum Institute in Copenhagen, which organized the campaign in Poland; he later became the Director General of the World Health Organization. At a Sunday luncheon meeting in a restaurant in Paris in December 1947, Holm proposed to Ludwic Rajchman, Chairman of the Executive Board of UNICEF, the launching of a bold and imaginative continent-wide tuberculosis campaign based on mass vaccination with BCG. Events moved rapidly, and in January Holm found himself directing a joint UNICEF and WHO tuberculosis control program for

Europe. BCG vaccination was an important part of that campaign. During the next three and one-half years, Holm's program tuberculin tested more than twenty-nine million European children and administered BCG vaccine to nearly fourteen million uninfected children in twenty-four countries. The program included not only Europe, but it also reached out to such remote sites as Sri Lanka and Ecuador. BCG was firmly established as a part of national tuberculosis control programs. Optimism ran high.

In 1947 the United States Public Health Service undertook to evaluate the potential usefulness of BCG vaccination for tuberculosis control in the United States. Muscogee County, Georgia was chosen as the test site. More than eleven thousand school children between five and nineteen years of age were enrolled in the study. All were tuberculin skin tested, and those who did not react were randomly assigned to receive BCG vaccine or a placebo. It soon became evident that almost all of the tuberculosis occurred in those persons who were already infected and had positive skin tests at the time the trial was initiated. No vaccine could offer these young persons protection. As for the uninfected children, five children who had been vaccinated developed tuberculosis, and three who were given placebo contracted the disease.[15] There was no protection offered by the vaccine, and BCG never gained widespread acceptance in the United States.

Georgina Feldberg has attempted to examine the American decision not to make BCG vaccination a part of its national campaign against tuberculosis.[16] Her thesis is that initial opposition by a few scientists critical of Calmette's statistical methods expanded in a climate of emphasis on social change as the over-riding need in tuberculosis control. Inflexibly, in her view, the American public health establishment "carved out a range of objections to BCG."[17] Feldberg appears to put aside the fact that those charged with designing tuberculosis control programs in the United States had data from their own well designed and carefully executed studies showing little protection. Surely, they must have felt that other measures of control would be more effective. Moreover, by the mid and late 1950s isoniazid prophylaxis was becoming an increasingly attractive tuberculosis control strategy (Chapter 25), and it was incompatible with widespread use of BCG.

Further trials of BCG were conducted in many countries. In some

BCG seemed to be effective, in others not. A well done study in Britain was particularly encouraging.[18] While there were still many experts who had reservations about BCG, acceptance of it grew. In May 1964 René Dubos, a distinguished microbiologist at the Rockefeller Institute in New York and a preeminent student of the tubercle bacillus, gave the prestigious J. Burns Amberson lecture to the American Thoracic Society. After acknowledging the deficiencies of the BCG preparations then available, Dubos assessed this vaccine as, "at present the one antibacterial vaccine for which evidence of activity in animals and man is the most impressive . . . "[19]

In the early 1960s the technique of freeze-drying was developed. Not only did this make available more tasty food for back-packers, it made available vaccines that did not need constant refrigeration. It did even more for BCG. Recall that Calmette and Guérin had altered the virulence of tubercle bacilli by repeatedly passing it from one culture to the next. Yet this same passage technique was the only means available of preserving the vaccine. In the four to five decades that had elapsed, it had become obvious that BCG produced in one laboratory looked very different from that produced in another laboratory. The mutational changes that had made BCG avirulent and useful as a vaccine had continued, small step by small step, during this long history of serial passage. Did these different looking vaccines also immunize differently? To this day, the answer to that question is not known.[20] The ability to freeze dry large "seed lots" of vaccine meant that repeated passage of cultures was no longer necessary. Production batches of vaccine could be grown starting with vials of a seed lot that had been stored for this purpose, and each vial would be identical with others from the same seed lot.

The World Health Organization has had a number of expert advisory committees, including one on tuberculosis. In December 1973 the WHO Expert Committee on Tuberculosis met in Geneva. The technical report of the deliberations of that meeting, the committee's Ninth Report, soon became the Bible and handbook for all concerned with tuberculosis control. This report laid out the essential blue print for tuberculosis control programs in a fashion that national health departments found applicable to their individual tuberculosis problems in the far-flung and diverse nations of the world. In that report the expert committee "emphasized that where infant tuberculosis is a problem, the widest possible coverage with BCG vaccination should be ensured as early in life as possible."[21] This challenge was met. In 1989 it was estimated that more than three billion doses had been given.[22] No other vaccine had been more widely used at that time.

The largest trial of BCG ever undertaken was begun in Chingleput in the Tamil Nandu district of South India in 1968. More than a quarter of a million persons were vaccinated, and as results began to roll in during the next two decades the world was dismayed to learn that BCG afforded no protection against tuberculosis in this largest of ever investigation.[23] However, Sriram Tripathy, who was Director of the Tuberculosis Research Centre in Madras that conducted the BCG trial and later became Director of the Indian Council of Medical Research, reanalyzed the data from that trial and cast a dissenting vote. He limited his analysis to those children who were clearly uninfected at the time of vaccination. Among them, overall protection was about seventeen percent, and in the six to ten year-old age group the protection was forty-five percent.[24]

The story of BCG has been one marked by enormous excitement alternating with great disappointment. Seventy-five years after its first use, we still do not know how effective it is. In an enormous undertaking, Graham Colditz and his colleagues from the Harvard School of Public Health undertook to reanalyze all of the information available. Their analysis suggested a protective efficacy of about fifty percent.[25] Taking a cynical position, one might look upon fifty percent as the halfway point between zero and one hundred percent! In the vaccine world, that leaves a lot of room for improvement.

In a very thoughtful review and analysis of BCG vaccine trials, George Comstock points out that most or all of the many studies conducted have met with problems, some potentially foreseeable, some not.[26] He points out that any attempt to use the tools of modern molecular medicine to achieve a new and perhaps better vaccine will have to accompanied by further field trials for vaccine evaluation. Hopefully, this problem can be approached with more success in the future than it has in the past.

Modern biomedical researchers continue to attack the problem of immunization against tuberculosis, and it may well be that the world will yet have an effective vaccine. Perhaps we will yet have a secure way of producing immunity to this devastating disease, of protecting poets like Keats, novelists like Charlotte Brontë, musicians like Frédéric Chopin, and the nearly three million unheralded persons who die of tuberculosis each year in our contemporary world.

16

Four Cornerposts of Science

When early settlers cleared the forests and broke the hard sod of North America, they built pole barns for the shelter of their animals and farm harvests. These barns were built not by framing walls on foundations but by erecting a series of poles or posts to which boards could be nailed and upon which a roof could be supported. Those barns were built post at a time, board after board, and shingle upon of shingle. So also is scientific knowledge acquired. The lives of Keats and Stevenson and the experiments of Lurie demonstrated that some individuals were more resistant to tuberculosis than others. Koch and then Calmette and Guérin showed that this resistance—immunity—could be induced by prior exposure to tubercle bacilli. Koch once more and Von Pirquet established that immune individuals reacted to soluble components, which we now term antigens, of cultures of tubercle bacilli. Thus, our scientific barn was built with the expanding knowledge of immunity to tuberculosis, immunity that plays an important role in determining the course of infection with the tubercle bacillus.

Let us now turn our attention to four more modern scientific discoveries that form the cornerposts of our current knowledge of the human body's capacity to become immune to the ravages of tuberculosis. These important bits of our knowledge should not be viewed alone, as isolated posts, for they are part of a structure with many posts, and none should belittle or ignore the enormous contributions of countless hundreds of other imaginative scientists who erected additional posts not described in this book. Rather, viewed in context, these four discoveries should be recognized as examples of parts—important parts—of the sheltering barn that protects our bodies from the ravages of windstorms of disease. Interestingly, it was curiosity-bred pursuit of scientific knowledge rather than a targeted inquiry into specific tuberculous disease processes that generated most our knowledge of these four cornerposts.

Merrill W. Chase erected the first post that we will consider. He was twenty-six years old in 1931 when he received the Ph.D. degree from Brown University for studies on toxins of an organism closely related to the one that causes typhoid fever. Studies of bacterial toxins were important at that time, for it was known that the serum or liquid, cell-free part of blood of immune individuals contained soluble antibodies that conferred protection against many such toxins. Koch's student, Emil von Behring, was awarded the first Nobel Prize given in medicine in 1901 for the discovery of antibodies to diphtheria toxin, and when the sled dog Balto and a series of heroic mushers carried antiserum against diphtheria toxin from Anchorage to Nome, Alaska over the Iditarod Trail in 1925, it was miracle-working protective antibodies that they carried.

1931 was not a prosperous time in this country, and Chase must have felt himself fortunate in the year following the award of his degree to have obtained a post as an assistant in the laboratory of Dr. Karl Landsteiner at the Rockefeller Institute in New York City. That institute, established in 1901 with an initial endowment gift from John D. Rockefeller of twenty thousand dollars, was a center of scientific excitement, and Karl Landsteiner was a famous immunologist who had discovered the ABO groups of human red blood cells. Landsteiner and John L. Jacobs, Chase's predecessor in the laboratory, were busy at work on the chemical nature of soluble antigens—substances that induce and elicite immune response—and they had chosen to use as their model the skin reactions of guinea pigs to two highly reactive chemicals, 2,4-dinitrochlorobenzene and picryl chloride (trinitrochlorobenzene). They thought these reactions provided a good model for human skin eczema.[1]

Merrill Chase's involvement with this field of study began in a substantial way in 1936. Initially, like Lurie, he tried to breed guinea pigs showing heightened reactivity to the chemicals. Later, learning of the findings of Jules Freund that certain components of tubercle bacilli heightened immune response to antigens, he began using tubercle bacilli to make his animals more responsive to the chemical agents.

In 1941, at the suggestion of Landsteiner, Chase was engaged in attempts to transfer the induced reactivity to chemical agents from one guinea pig to another. Serum from sensitized animals did not transfer reactivity, even though the serum was shown to contain antibodies to the chemical agents. Chase then tried using extracts of skin. Later, seeking more abundant material, he used washings from the abdominal peritoneal cavities of animals he had sensitized not in the skin but in the peritoneum. These transfers were successful. Chase then centrifuged the material from the guinea pig peritoneal exudates and found that the clarified fluid of these exudates did not transfer immunity but that the cells in the fluid did. Chase examined these cells under a microscope. They were uniformly white blood cells of a type we term lymphocytes. Chase had demonstrated that the capacity to transfer the immune reactions he studied rested with and only with lymphocytes.

Merrill Chase proudly showed his centrifuged cells to his mentor, Karl Landsteiner. The famous man was delighted with his assistant's elegant work, but stated that the transfer was certainly due to cell-fixed antibodies, not the lymphocytes Chase observed. Chase thought otherwise, but he did not argue with the famous man. History, however, proved Chase correct and Landsteiner in error. Lymphocytes are the key cells responsible for skin eczema and also for the immune responses that determine the pathogenesis of tuberculosis. Antibodies, cell-fixed or other, have nothing to do with the type of reactions that Chase was studying and that mediate immunity to tuberculosis.

In 1943, following Landsteiner's death, Merrill Chase moved to the laboratory of René J. Dubos, still at the Rockefeller Institute. Dubos was interested in tuberculosis and encouraged Chase to extend his studies to reactions to tuberculin. This he did, and in 1945 he reported the transfer of tuberculin reactions in guinea pigs using washed lymphocytes.[2]

The skin reactions that Chase studied had the characteristic feature of being delayed in onset. That is, the reactions in the animals' skin did not begin immediately and needed two to three days to develop fully. As anyone who has experienced the skin reaction to poison ivy knows, there are many such delayed hypersensitivity reactions, and tuberculin skin reactions such as those first studied by von Pirquet are among them. This feature has led to the sobriquet "delayed hypersensitivity" for these lymphocyte-mediated immune responses.

To Merrill Chase goes the credit for first demonstrating and recognizing the central role of lymphocytes in cellular immunity and for erecting the first of our four cornerposts. In the later years of his long career, Chase engaged in many studies of immunity to tuberculosis. But his seminal discoveries were made in the context of the study of eczema. Had Karl Landsteiner been a student of tuberculosis, history might have been written differently. By 1904 Maragliano in Italy had described an antibody-containing antiserum for tuberculosis, and during the following two years it was used to treat patients at the Phipps Institute in Philadelphia. The results were disappointing, and Chase's work explained why. It was clear that antibodies did not mediate immune resistance to tuberculosis in those patients.[3]

We must now leap ahead two decades. The next cornerpost to be considered cannot be attributed to a single individual but rather to a small number of highly imaginative scientists interested in lymphocyte-mediated, delayed hypersensitivity reactions. Tuberculin reactions had come to be recognized as a paradigm for these reactions, and tuberculin was easily at hand for their study. In fact, the work of Florence Seibert described in Chapter 13 had made her purified protein derivative (PPD) of tuberculin readily available. The stage was set for further investigations of the mechanism of immunity to tuberculosis.

In New Zealand, Professors G. Permain, R.R. Lycette, and P.H. Fitzgerald had been studying cellular reactions to materials extracted from plants. When lymphocytes were incubated together with the plant materials, they changed their form to a more primitive one. The Kiwi investigators then substituted tuberculin for the plant extract. When and only when the lymphocytes came from a tuberculin-immune animal, similar changes in the cell morphology occurred.[4] At the same time and working totally independently in Chicago, Robert Schrek performed almost identical experiments and found almost identical results.[5] A few years later, C.F. "Fritz" Hinz and I demonstrated that this cell reaction correlated quantitatively with tuberculin skin test reactions in tuberculin-sensitive persons.[6] Here was a reaction that not only confirmed the importance of lymphocytes in tuberculin immunity but that greatly facilitated the laboratory study of tuberculin immunity. It was now possible to study tuberculin reactions not only in the skin of the sensitized individual but in bench top laboratory experiments.

Among other observations concerning the reaction of peritoneal exudate cells from immune animals to tuberculin, it had been noted that tuberculin inhibited the migration of these cells across a glass surface.

Crude cell preparations were used to demonstrate this phenomenon, and in these preparations it appeared to be a type of scavenger cell named a macrophage, not the lymphocyte, that was the mobile migrant. Once again, two laboratories investigating cellular immune mechanisms independently turned their attention to the same problem. Drs. John R. David,[7] at New York University, and Barry R. Bloom and Boyce Bennet,[8] at Albert Einstein College of Medicine, both in New York City, studied the migration of macrophages and found that the macrophages could come from any animal but that inhibition of migration was produced only when lymphocytes from a tuberculin-sensitive animal were added to the culture. Indeed, the whole lymphocyte was not necessary. What was needed was a soluble substance secreted by the lymphocyte. That is, immune lymphocytes communicated with other cells—macrophages—by means of a soluble messenger substance produced by the lymphocytes in response to stimulation with tuberculin. This substance became known as MIF—macrophage inhibition factor. Over the ensuing decades, many such antigen-induced, soluble mediators of immune responses have been discovered, and they have come to be known as lymphokines, when produced only by lymphocytes, or more generally as cytokines.

This then is our second cornerpost—a mechanism by which immune lymphocytes communicate with other cells to direct the complex cellular reactions that protect immune persons from tuberculosis. The mechanism is specific, for lymphocytes produce their soluble mediators only when stimulated by antigens. Two of those persons who erected this cornerpost have gone on to distinguished immunology research careers, John David at Harvard, where he has studied not only tuberculosis but also parasitic diseases, and Barry Bloom at Albert Einstein College of Medicine, where he has studied the immunology of tuberculosis and also leprosy, a disease produced by a bacillus closely related to the tubercle bacillus.

The science of immunology moved rapidly to erect a third cornerpost. The leading and central role was taken by Dr. Robert A. Good, a pediatrician at the University of Minnesota. Good was not interested in tuberculosis. Rather, he was interested in children who were born with deficient immune systems, children whom some doctors tried to protect by isolating in plastic bubbles to the delight of the tabloid sensationalist press. Good noted that these children were not all the same.

Some children were susceptible to some infections, some to others, and Good thought of these differences in susceptibility as experiments of nature. To Good it was clear that there was not a single protective immune system but at least two separate immune systems.[9]

In 1952 Good and a colleague, Richard Varco, encountered a patient with a defect in delayed hypersensitivity and cellular immunity in association with a tumor of the thymus gland. In 1956 Bruce Glick had discovered that chickens who had had a hind gut-derived organ called the bursa of Fabricius removed as young chicks were unable to produce antibody. His report of his discovery was turned down by the leading research journal *Science* and appeared in *Poultry Science*, where it attracted little attention from immunologists. Taken together, these observations meant that there were separate situations of immunodeficiency. One, a defect in cellular, delayed immunity, appeared to be related to the thymus; the other, a defect in antibody production, appeared to be related to the bursa of Fabricius in chickens and the bone marrow in humans. Good recognized this dichotomy.

During the 1960s a great deal was learned about these two immune systems. Both were dependent upon lymphocytes, and both classes of lymphocytes looked the same under the microscope. However, their cell surfaces were not the same, and tools and methods for sorting them out were developed. The antibody-related lymphocytes came to be called B-lymphocytes or simply B-cells, recognizing their relationship to the bursa of the chicken. The lymphocytes controlling delayed hypersensitivity came to be called T-lymphocytes or T-cells because of their association with the thymus gland.

Biology is complex. Good's neat classification of lymphocytes into B- and T-cells soon gave way to further classification as it became apparent that there are many distinct types of T-lymphocytes with different functions. They can be identified by features of their cell surfaces. One group of T-lymphocytes, known as CD4$^+$ cells appears to be the master of the lymphocyte pack, retaining immunologic memory and secreting cytokines to direct the activity of other cells in the immune system—the maestro of an incredibly complex symphony orchestra. So it is that the third cornerpost includes not only the recognition of a dual immune system but also a mechanism of control based upon a cell responsible for immunologic memory.

The final cornerpost of our immunologic barn was erected by Kenneth S. Warren, a scientist at Case Western Reserve University in Cleveland. Warren, at the urging to his former Harvard teacher Thomas Weller, followed his medical school and internship training with travel to Brazil and St. Lucia, where he studied schistosomiasis, the disease known as bilharzia to British colonialists of the nineteenth century. While working at the Rockefeller Foundation research station in St. Lucia, Warren began infecting mice with bilharzia parasites, and in so doing he developed an animal model for this disease that permitted him to study its pathogenesis. When Warren left St. Lucia, he moved to Cleveland, and there he began his seminal studies of the immunology of schistosomiasis.[10]

Warren knew that the tissue response to the invading eggs of the schistosomiasis parasite was an organized aggregation of immune cells in the tissue and surrounding the egg. The resulting tissue lesion was of a type known as a granuloma. He believed this granuloma was essentially similar to the granulomas called tubercula by Hippocrates and known since the time of Laennec and Koch to surround tubercle bacilli in human tissues. The noted pathologist and student of tuberculosis Arnold Rich had considered these granulomas to be a nonspecific response of the body to an alien material, but Warren wondered if this response was not mediated by cellular immune mechanisms. Irwin Lepow, one of Warren's faculty colleagues in Cleveland, challenged him to test his ideas. It would be necessary, Lepow suggested, to demonstrate (1) that the capacity to form granulomas in response to the eggs correlated with other manifestations of delayed hypersensitivity, (2) that it could be transferred by immune lymphocytes, and (3) that it was absent in animals deficient of these cells. Warren accepted the challenge and began an elegant set of experiments.

Warren used his mouse model for his studies in Cleveland. Large fish tanks were used to grow snails, which carry the parasite. Mice lived in cages and were infected by dipping their tails into water containing the bilharzia larvae. Special instruments were obtained to measure the size of granulomas seen when tissues from the infected mice were studied under the microscope. In logical sequence, one observation followed another. Lepow's criteria were met. Granuloma size was found to correlate with skin reactivity to schistosome extract. The ability to form granulomas in response to schistosome eggs was transferred from an immune animal to a naive animal by lymphocytes but not serum. The capacity to respond to schistosome eggs with granuloma formation was abolished by removing the thymus gland of newborn mice. Studies of chicks with the bursa removed were less conclusive because chickens provided a poor model for schistosomiasis.[11]

Warren and his colleagues went a step further. They purified a soluble antigen from schistosome eggs and then coated the surface of bentonite clay particles about the size of the eggs with this antigen. When injected into immune mice, granulomas formed. Clearly, the immune response was directed at soluble antigens, not entire eggs. It was a logical extension from this work to coat similarly small bentonite particles with tuberculin. These coated particles elicited granulomas in mice hypersensitive to tubercle bacilli.[12] The fourth cornerpost was in place—the discovery that the formation of granulomas or tubercles is an immunologically-mediated event.

Kenneth Warren continued his interest in parasitic diseases, especially schistosomiasis. He moved from his laboratory in Cleveland to the Rockefeller Foundation to be come its Vice President for Medical Affairs. In this position he supported research on parasitic diseases in many laboratories throughout the world.

The body of a person infected with tubercle bacilli responds to this invader by mobilizing an immune system that is elegant in its specificity and complex in its action. Many cells are involved, under the control of CD4+ T-lymphocytes that secrete cytokines that direct other cells to form granulomas and carry out other immunologic processes. This complex immune system produces resistance to infection and defends the body against the invasion of the tubercle bacillus. As we have learned earlier, this defense is usually effective. The disease that we call tuberculosis and that our forbearers called consumption occurs when it is not.

17

The Cursed Duet

In the last chapter, we learned of the CD4+ T-lymphocyte, the master of the lymphocyte pack, the maestro of an incredibly complex symphony orchestra. When a talented musician gives a solo recital, no conductor is needed. When a string quartet puts bows to strings to perform one of Beethoven's masterpieces, a nod of a head suffices to start the music, and the performers rely on their collective ears to coordinate their music. However, large symphony orchestras need a maestro. They simply do not function well without a conductor. The same is true of immune systems. Without CD4+ T-lymphocytes, the immune system cannot function and cannot protect us from tuberculosis.

In 1959 a twenty-five year-old British merchant seaman died in Manchester, England.[1] His illness puzzled his physicians. He wasted of a consumptive disease, and his doctors treated him for tuberculosis, although they were not able to establish that diagnosis. This treatment did not help him. He went on to develop other pulmonary infections, rare infections, infections known only to occur in persons whose immune systems had been severely damaged. In 1970 preserved tissues from the ill-fated sailor were examined by modern DNA fingerprinting techniques and found to contain remnants of the virus that causes AIDS, the acquired immunodeficiency syndrome. This virus, unknown to medical science at the time, caused his death.

More than twenty years later, in 1981, the United States Centers for Disease Control received five reports of young American men with rare pulmonary infections.[2] All of these men were homosexuals. Then more cases were reported, not only in homosexual men, but in immigrants from Haiti, in patients with hemophilia, and intravenous drug users. It soon became painfully apparent that America was dealing with an epidemic of a new and fatal disease. An enormous effort, centered initially at the Centers for Disease control in Atlanta, Georgia and at the National Institutes of Health in Bethesda, Maryland but soon extending to academic research laboratories throughout the world, identified the new disease as due to a virus, the human immunodeficiency virus (HIV). Within an amazingly short decade, AIDS—acquired immunodeficiency syndrome—was recognized, its cause identified, its epidemiology and pathogenesis unravelled, new diagnostic tests developed, and trials initiated of newly developed drugs for treatment. As part of this explosion of information, scientists developed the techniques that permitted the retrospective diagnosis of AIDS in the British sailor who died in 1959.

The new knowledge made one fact abundantly clear. This new human immunodeficiency virus—HIV—has as its primary target the $CD4^+$ T-lymphocyte, the maestro of the immune system, and once it infects these cells, it ultimately destroys them. Other cells of the body, including macrophages, are also attacked, but the awesome aspect of AIDS is that its victims are left without effective immunity, defenseless against many infections, prominently including tuberculosis. Of course, antibiotics and other drugs may be used to treat infections in AIDS patients, but with variable success in the absence of the body's immune responses.

Meanwhile, the epidemic in the United States exploded. By February 1983, one thousand cases had been reported. By August 1983, two thousand. By October 1995, five hundred thousand. Unfortunately, no means of aborting the epidemic, of protecting uninfected persons, or of curing the disease have yet been found.

David Serwadda was the District Medical Officer in the Rakai district of southwestern Uganda in the early 1980s. An epidemic of a disease called "slim disease" by the local residents was in full swing. Young men and women wasted and died. Serwadda was struck by the resemblance of the illness he witnessed to the newly described entity of AIDS. He enlisted the help of colleagues from the Makerere University Faculty of Medicine in Kampala, Uganda and of British scientists. Together they investigated this epidemic and reported their findings in the international journal, Lancet.[3] Slim disease was AIDS. This new killer was not just a disease of North American men and Haitians but also of Africans. In fact, studies of blood samples collected in Uganda in 1972 and 1973 and saved since made it evident that the disease was already established there by the early 1970s. By the mid 1990s, some ten or twelve percent of all Ugandans were infected with the AIDS virus, and in young adult populations the figure reached thirty to forty percent. African men and women are equally afflicted by this lethal disease, and in Africa the route of transmission is almost exclusively sexual.

Drs. Gnana Sunderam, Lee Reichman, and their colleagues working in the Pulmonary Disease Division at the New Jersey Medical School University Hospital in Newark, New Jersey noted that twenty-nine of one hundred and thirty-six adults with AIDS seen at their hospital between 1981 and 1985 had developed tuberculosis.[4] Their tuberculosis was more severe and more rapidly progressive than the New Jersey doctors were accustomed to seeing in nonAIDS patients. Moreover, the clinical features of tuberculosis in these patients were often unusual. They suggested that tuberculosis should be considered a complication of AIDS. Drs. Arthur Pitchenik and Howard Rubinson reported a similar situation among their Haitian AIDS patients in Florida,[5] and soon hospitals throughout America found themselves dealing not only with AIDS but with fulminant tuberculosis accompanying AIDS.

Dr. Richard Goodgame was working as a Baptist missionary in Kampala, Uganda. Throughout many war-torn years, he labored at Makerere University School of Medicine and Mulago Hospital, struggling to keep medical education alive in the face of the anti-intellectual and genocidal rule of Idi Amin. AIDS patients swamped the hospital service on which he worked, and most of them had tuberculosis as well. In his words, "tuberculosis is ubiquitous."[6]

Sunderam, Reichman, and their colleagues were correct when they first reported that tuberculosis was different in AIDS patients from normal persons.[7] The disease tends to spread beyond the lungs, and involve lymph nodes and other parts of the body. In the lungs the presentations of tuberculosis are more acute than they are in normal persons. The slowly progressive or chronic courses that were vividly seen in the cases of Frédéric Chopin and Robert Louis Stevenson simply do not occur in AIDS patients. Fulminant tuberculous pneumonias occur. Even with modern drug treatment, many AIDS patients with tuberculosis die.

Neither AIDS nor tuberculosis can occur in an individual unless that person is infected with the AIDS virus or the tuberculosis bacillus. However, when a person is infected with both germs, then the extraor-

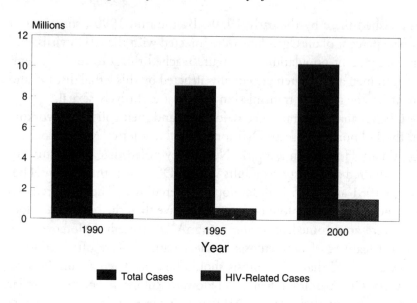

Figure 17.1. Projected total number of cases of tuberculosis and number of HIV-related cases in the world from 1990 to 2000. Both the total number and the number of HIV-related cases are expected to increase. Data from Dolin PJ, Raviglione MC, Kochi A. Global tuberculosis incidence and mortality during 1990-2000. Bull World Health Org 1994; 72:213-20.

dinary synergism of these two killers moves to the fore. "The cursed duet," said Professor Jacques Chrétien.[8] As we noted in Chapter 6, the tubercle bacillus infects about one-third of the population of the world. Small wonder, then that tuberculosis is the number one infection in the world for AIDS patients. Moreover, the situation is clearly going to get worse. Working with data reported to the World Health Organization, Dolin and his colleagues have estimated that the incidence of tuberculosis in the world will increase during the decade from 1990 to 2000 from seven and one-half million to ten million, two hundred thousand cases annually, an increase of thirty-five percent.[9] The number of HIV-related cases will also increase and will represent about fourteen percent of the total. These projections are shown in Figure 17.1.

The susceptibility of AIDS patients extends beyond the tubercle bacillus to one of its cousins. *Mycobacterium avium* is related to the tubercle bacillus in the same way that a tiger is related to a pussy cat—same genus, different species. *M. avium*, first isolated from a bird—hence its name—is a ubiquitous water and soil resident, to which everyone is exposed. It is not killed by chlorination, and is present in our drinking water. It is a pussy cat; it does not produce disease in most of us. But it causes disease of many organs in AIDS patients late in their illness when their CD4$^+$ cells have dropped to almost zero. In those persons, *M. avium* is a tiger.

Dr. Robert Good looked upon the immunodeficiencies of the children under his care as experiments of nature, experiments that led him to ask why some children with some defects developed certain infections while others developed other diseases, experiments that ultimately permitted him to recognize the presence of two separate immune systems. The awful experiment of AIDS similarly points out the singular role of CD4$^+$ T-lymphocytes in protecting us from tuberculosis. The keystone of the body's defense against tuberculosis is destroyed by the AIDS virus, and without it the immune system that protects us against tuberculosis cannot function. The combination of HIV and *M. tuberculosis* is, indeed, a cursed duet.

PART IV

Magic Mountains and Magic Bullets
The Treatment of Tuberculosis

Christopher Robin
Had wheezles
And sneezles
They bundled him
Into
His bed, . . .
They sent for some doctors
In sneezles
And wheezles
To tell them what ought
To be done. . . .
They said "If he freezles
In draughts and in breezles
Then PHTHEEZLES
May even ensue."
A. A. Milne[1]

18

Victories

As we begin our consideration of the attempts—some more successful than others—that the medical profession has made to treat tuberculosis, we might do well to reflect on the stories of two women who battled this disease and conquered it. They fought their battles apart from the medical establishment and its armamentarium of nostrums. That they emerged victorious tells us that the captain of death is not the victor in every conflict.

Alice Marble was a remarkable woman. A feisty tom-boy who grew into a strikingly beautiful woman. A friend of the rich and famous, and close confidante of some of Hollywood's most glamorous stars. A frequent guest of millionaires William Randolph Hearst and Will Dupont. A sometimes night club singer. A spy for American army intelligence during World War II. Above all, the most outstanding woman tennis player of the 1930s. Four times winner of the national women's singles championship (United States Open) at Forest Hills; winner of the last prewar women's singles world championship at Wimbleton in 1939; the number one ranked woman player from 1936 through 1940. And a victim of tuberculosis.[2]

Alice Marble sailed to France on the German liner *Bremen* in May of 1934 to play in a series of matches leading up to the Wightman Cup competition in June at Wimbledon. She arrived at Le Havre feeling tired with pains in her chest and back. Her team-mates arranged for her to see a doctor, who told her she was anemic. She had trouble sleeping. Nevertheless, she pulled herself together and prepared to play her matches.

In the first set of her opening match against Sylvia Henrotin, France's second ranked woman player, Alice Marble was down five games to one. She felt dizzy and short of breath. Playing took every bit of her will power. She missed her first two serves. The score was love-fifteen. She raised her racquet to serve again and collapsed onto the clay, to be carried off the court. The beautiful athletic young woman, pride of America's tennis world, had pleurisy due to tuberculosis. "I'm sorry," her doctor told her, "but you will never be strong enough to play tennis again."

Alice returned home to the United States. Her coach and close companion, Eleanor "Teach" Tennant, met her in New York and accompanied her across the country to her home in San Francisco. Carried into her family's house by her brothers, she was settled into an upstairs bedroom to begin the rest that she hoped would bring a return of her life. Soon she moved, for Teach arranged for her to be admitted to Pottenger's Sanatorium in Monrovia, California. There, she settled into her confined life in one of the sanatorium's cottages.

> "I was under orders to stay in bed except to go to the bathroom. The nurses (guards, I called them) came by the cottage frequently to make sure I complied. One day they found me gone. After a search, two white-clad Amazons came panting up to where I sat on the bank of the lake. I was puffing calmly on a cigarette.
>
> "One of them snatched it from my lips. 'You're not supposed to smoke!'
>
> "'I don't.' I stood up and walked back to the cabin, pleased in a perverse way that I had created a stir. The place was deadly dull, filled with people like me, vegetating."

Weeks stretched on to months. There seemed to be no end to the confinement to which Dr. Pottenger sentenced Alice.

> "'The doctor says you're doing fine, but you need another six weeks of rest,' Teach said. I glared at Pottinger [sic], who nodded."

Boredom, restlessness, and anxiety ultimately gave way to despair. Then, one day, a letter arrived that was to change Alice's attitude towards her illness. "Dear Alice. You don't know me, but your tennis teacher is also my teacher, and she has told me all about you," the letter began. The letter told of the writer's battle to recover from an automobile accident that threatened to destroy her acting career. "Well, I proved the doctors wrong. I made my career come true, just as you can—if you'll fight," the letter continued. The letter was from Carole Lombard, Hollywood's reigning beauty. The letter struck a finely-tuned chime in Alice's heart, and she responded. She began her fight. The letter also initiated a close friendship that continued until Carole Lombard's tragic death in an aviation disaster.

Alice Marble picked herself up and walked out of Dr. Pottenger's sanatorium. As she described the episode,

> "I was tired of people telling me what I *couldn't* do. My six-week stay had turned into eight months. . . . The doctor had finally given me permission to spend fifteen minutes a day outside, and to walk to the pond seventy-five feet away. This wasn't living! It wasn't me! When Teach came to visit, my bags were packed.
>
> "'I'm never going to get well here,' I told her. 'If I stay much longer, I'll never get out of here alive. I've got to do it now.'
>
> "She looked at me, gauging the determination in my eyes. 'If you can make it to the car, we'll leave right now.'
>
> "'I'll make it to the car.' None of my clothes fit, so I threw a coat over my pajamas and picked up my bag."

Marble's strength returned slowly, but within a few months she was again playing tennis and playing well. In 1936, two years after her collapse, she won the United States women's singles, women's doubles, and mixed doubles championships at Forest Hills. She went on to repeated tennis conquests, her victories interrupted only by World War II. At the end of the war, she was enlisted as a spy by American army intelligence, and collected information on Nazi bank accounts in Switzerland from a former lover. In her later years Alice Marble taught, coached, and sponsored many of the new generation of aggressive women tennis players of the second half of the twentieth century. She died in 1990 at the age of seventy-seven, never again having experienced tuberculosis.

Towards the end of his career, Dr. Francis Marion Pottenger, the physician who treated Alice Marble, wrote a comprehensive textbook on tuberculosis.[3] The book was published in 1948, just at the time when effective drug treatment of tuberculosis was arriving on the medical scene and rendering obsolete the forms of treatment Pottenger espoused. The book, Pottenger explains in his preface was based on his fifty years of clinical practice. Let us see what he wrote about the treatment of tuberculosis. It may give us insights as to how he viewed his famous athlete patient.

"The properly conducted sanatorium," Pottenger wrote, "is truly a haven of rest for the tuberculous patient. It separates him from the bustling world without, and gives him rest of mind and rest of body. It shields him from the cares and responsibilities of home and business; it protects him from his friends and limits the demands made upon his energy. It is appreciated by the ill patient when he first enters the institution, but, alas, is too often forgotten when he feels better and tires of the isolation and inactivity, which are such important factors in cure, and desires to go home."[4] It would not have surprised Alice Marble to have read that statement of the philosophy that guided Pottenger's management of his patients. It embodied everything against which she rebelled.

Judging from the statements made by Alice Marble in her autobiography,[5] the form of tuberculosis she suffered was almost certainly pleurisy with effusion. This form of disease is an early form with a relatively good near-term outlook, with or without treatment. What does Pottenger say of treating this form of disease? "The patient should be put to bed in the open air and kept warm." He goes on to conclude his discussion by stating, "all of the measures which are useful in treating the underlying tuberculosis should be rigidly carried out in all tuberculous patients no matter what the complication on the part of the pleura."[6] Whether because her form of tuberculosis was a mild one, because of her indomitable spirit, or because of good luck, Alice Marble won her victory over tuberculosis despite rather than because of the ministrations of Dr. Pottenger.

While Alice Marble was chalking up victory after victory on the tennis court, Josephine Baker was claiming victory over the world's entertainment courts.[7] Born in the abject poverty of a shanty town in Saint Louis, Josephine Baker found in her love of the stage and her ability to dance an escape to a better life. Initially a comedy star, then a dancer, and finally a singer, she rose to her greatest fame in France. Strikingly beautiful, her most famous venue was the Folies-Bergère, where she opened her appearances in lavish costumes and closed by dancing wearing only a bunch of bananas strung about her waist.

Baker toured throughout Europe, North Africa, and South America, performing for the rich and famous and becoming rich and famous herself; she was adored by royalty. However, she exiled herself from the

United States, unwilling to return to a land of racial prejudice after France had opened its doors and hearts to her without thinking of her skin color. She became a French citizen.

World War II erupted in Europe. France fell to the Nazis. Northern France was occupied by German troops; southern France ruled by a puppet government in Vichy. Free French resistance fighters, held together by the leadership of General Charles de Gaulle, fled to Algiers to set up a government in exile. Josephine Baker thought of it as a phony war, for it seemed to have little impact on her theatrical world. Then, French intelligence officers approached her and asked her to act as a secret courier. Her ability to move freely across Europe was of great value to them. Josephine Baker had no hesitation in accepting.

Josephine Baker was ready to go to North Africa, where she had performed before and where she could easily continue her career as cover for her espionage activities. However, she had to find a way to break her contract for performances in Marseilles. She had had a dreadful cough for several months, and she felt that a medical examination might lead to a credible recommendation for a warmer climate that would allow her to escape from the clauses of her contract. She consulted a physician. The news was more than she expected. Yes, she would do well to go to North Africa, for she had tuberculosis in both lungs.

For the next two years, Josephine Baker battled illness. Her autobiography gives few details of her disease; there were other things more important in her life. She does not appear to have received any treatment directed at tuberculosis, nor does she describe care at any specialized facility.[8] During this time she traveled frequently to Portugal to perform in that neutral country whose capital, Lisbon, was a major espionage center. Her music went with her, covered in invisible ink with information gathered by French resistance fighters. She also entertained Allied troops as they fought to regain Africa from the troops of German General Rommel. Following the war, Josephine Baker's heroism was recognized. Sublieutenant Baker was made Chevalier of the Legion of Honor.

Following the return of peace to Europe and the world, Josephine Baker resumed her career on the stage. Her tuberculosis was behind her, and it did not recur. She was repeatedly invited to perform in the United States, always refusing because racial discrimination excluded her own people from her audiences. Finally, the barrier came down at a triumphant performance in Miami. With that, she joined the crusade for desegregation in the United States, tirelessly devoting herself to this cause. Together with her third husband, musician Jo Bouillon, Josephine Baker, whose two pregnancies had ended in miscarriages, began adopting orphaned children of many races, ultimately bringing together at her French chateau a "rainbow tribe" of twelve children whose lives together she felt provided a model of racial harmony for the world. Josephine Baker died in 1975, at the age of sixty-eight, a few days after a triumphant come-back performance in Paris. She had suffered repeated heart attacks; her final curtain was apparently brought down by a stroke.

Alice Marble and Josephine Baker, two remarkable women with lives that paralleled one another in many ways. Both fought the good fight, finished the race, kept the faith. Both conquered tuberculosis, and both did it without the help of or perhaps in spite of the aid of their doctors. Were their victories unique? Does anyone recover from this awful disease without treatment? Before we consider the accomplishments of modern treatment, we need to answer that question.

Stefan Grzybowski is a great bear of a man. He is jovial and fun loving, a witty raconteur. He is also the owner of a sharply honed mind, and he has used his mind to study tuberculosis. A Polish emigrant to Vancouver, Canada, he has looked at tuberculosis from the vantage point of an international citizen willing to question and challenge dogma from any source. Among his many contributions has been an effort to answer the question of what happens to people with untreated tuberculosis. Together with his student and younger colleague, Donald Enarson, Stefan Grzybowski searched out and analyzed reports of the outcome of tuberculosis in patients from various parts of the world in the era before modern drug treatment.[9] Over the five years following the recognition of tuberculosis, about half of the disease's victims die. About one in five consumptives remains chronically ill. And there is a fortunate quarter to one-third of tuberculosis patients that recovers good health. Alice Marble and Josephine Baker were among the fortunate. The miracle of modern drug treatment is that it makes this good fortune available to all.

19

Wolf's Liver and Sea Voyages

What we expect of a physician and of medical treatment is conditioned by what we expect of our illness. When we seek treatment for pneumonia, we expect an antibiotic to bring cure and return to normal health. When we have cancer, we hope that surgery and chemotherapy may result in a cure or, if not, at least a respite from the disease. When we have a common cold, we hope that remedies from the long shelves of the local pharmacy will bring some relief while we endure the affliction. As for tuberculosis, we are confident that modern treatment will cure us, although we may recognize that successful therapy may take more time than it does for other infections. These expectations are related to our understanding of these diseases. Pneumonia and tuberculosis are caused by well understood germs, for which we have magic bullets—drugs that will kill the germs but do us no harm. The common cold is caused by a virus, for which there currently is no curative agent. Cancer is a bit more shadowy. We are not sure what causes it, despite having a pretty good understanding of its nature, and we are not sure just what the surgeon's scalpel or the oncologist's chemotherapy can accomplish.

So what must people of previous times who had little understanding of illness have expected of their physicians and the treatment they offered? What did they hope for in the treatment of consumption? Not surprisingly, expectations of medical treatment have varied as have the treatments themselves as human perceptions of the causation of illness have evolved.

For early people ill health, including consumption, represented the expression of displeasure of not always benevolent gods, and the roles of physicians and priests were intertwined. In the twenty-eighth chapter of Deuteronomy, Moses cautions the Israelites that if they do not obey the voice of the Lord their God, then "the Lord will smite you with consumption." In the New Testament, in Chapter 9 of the Book of John, Jesus and his disciples meet a man blind from his birth. "Who sinned", the disciples ask, "this man or his parents, that he was born blind?" In the fifth century, St. Augustine taught that all diseases were due to demons. As we have seen in Chapter 3, about the time of St. Augustine, European royalty first claimed to be able to cure scrofula—tuberculosis of the lymph glands of the neck—by touching. This form of treatment was, in fact, a form of exorcism. It was espoused by the Church, and it became codified in Christian liturgy.

Some of the belief in the mystical, satanic, or divine origins of disease persisted into more modern times. In nineteenth century New England, some thought that those who died of tuberculosis were able to return as vampires and cause the wasting of their consumptive victims.[1] Bodies of the tuberculous dead were exhumed, so that the heart could be burned. An eighteenth century skeleton from a Connecticut grave exposed in 1990 by eroding sand and gravel was found to have pathological evidence of tuberculosis. The long thigh bones had evidently been rearranged at some time after the original burial to form a cross over the body's chest. In 1854, a Connecticut newspaper, the *Norwich Courier* described the exhumation and burning of the body of man who had died eight years previously of tuberculosis because two of his sons had become victims of the same disease.[2]

As thought evolved and less mystical and more ordinary explanations were sought for the cause of illness, the people of early classical civilizations came to think of disease as resulting from evil humors within the body. Therapies based on removing these malevolent substances from the body developed and persisted until the dawning of microbiology made it apparent that specific microorganisms caused infectious diseases. Sweating, urinating, and defecating were thought to be methods of cleansing the body, and treatment that promoted these bodily functions were widely used for many diseases, including tuberculosis. Blood letting was a logical extension, and leeches were applied to suck blood from patients. Indeed, doctors came to be called leeches colloquially. As we saw in Chapter 7, Chopin was horrified by the use of blood letting and blistering agents in the treatment of his sister. Again in Chapter 12, we noted that his physician bled the dying poet Keats. Morton's *Phthisiologia*, perhaps the most widely read text on tuberculosis of its day, recommended blood letting in 1689 "to prevent the hectic and colliquative heat or catarrhous state of the blood, or at least lessen it." While it was thought that "bleeding may do mischief in confirmed consumption," it was recommended as "very beneficial in the beginning."[3] This text also recommended the use of emetics to induce vomiting, cathartics and diuretics, and heat to induce sweating.

A more enlightened approach to the treatment of tuberculosis appears to have arisen with the ancient Greeks. They recommended measures intended to improve the patient's general health and strengthen bodily resistance to tuberculosis. Prescriptions commonly included milk, mild exercise, and warm climates. Pliny the Elder wrote, "For phthisis one has the liver of the wolf in wine, the lard of a thin sow fed on herbs, the flesh of an ass with a bouillon made from it . . . a drink from the shavings of the hoof of the ox scalded with honey . . . ashes of the tongues of pigs in wine or dried rosin with the lung of the deer, especially the short-horned deer, dried and steamed and powdered in wine."[4] The concept of a tonic to general health clearly underlies the thinking behind this pharmacopeia.

Milk has enjoyed an enduring place as a health-promoting tonic in the treatment of tuberculosis. Galen recommended it. At the turn of the fourteenth century, John of Gaddesden published *Rosa Angelica Practica Medicina a Capite ad Pedes*. This "head to toe" medical text was cited by Chaucer as one of the most widely used medical books of the era. For tuberculosis it prescribes, "As to food, the best is the milk of a young brunette with her first child, which should be a boy; the young woman should be well favored and should eat and drink in moderation. Failing a wet nurse, the milk of other animals might be used in the following order of choice: the ass, the goat, and the cow."[5] In 1903, at the dawning of a more rational approach to the treatment of tuberculosis, a patient of Lawrence Francis Flick wrote to the distinguished tuberculosis physician, "I am able to keep up the sixteen glasses of milk and twelve eggs per day . . ."[6] At the Pottenger Sanatorium, where Alice Marble sought cure, milk was served at every meal. "Pasteurization and other heat processing of milk," wrote Dr. Pottenger without basis in fact, "interferes with the assimilation of calcium and the proper utilization of milk as a food. Therefore, raw milk is preferable if the supply comes from a healthy herd, and the milk is produced in a cleanly manner."[7]

Throughout history, physicians have recommended and patients sought salubrious climates for the cure of consumption. Which climates have been considered most healthy? There has been a substantial range of expert medical opinion. In classical times, Celsus and Galen recommended warm climates.[8] As we have seen, Chopin, Keats, and Stevenson all sought the balmier weather of the Mediterranean Riviera. However, more modern medicine has demanded a more austere climate for the treatment of tuberculosis. In 1840, the London physician George Bodington wrote. "Sharp frosty days in the winter season are most favorable. The application of cold pure air to the interior surface of the lungs is the most powerful sedative that can be applied."[9] William Osler, dean of American physicians of his era and perhaps the most famous professor of medicine in American history, wrote in 1900 that, "for more than two centuries the clearer-headed members of the profession have known that an open air life sometimes cures a case of phthisis." Open air schools became popular for tuberculous children in the early twentieth century. "As it was popularly described by open-air school advocates," reports historian Richard A. Meckel, "[the] regimen basically consisted of the provision of 'double rations of air, double rations of food, and half rations of work.'"[10] All readers of Thomas Mann's classic novel *Magic Mountain* remember the ritualistic wrapping in blankets of Hans Castorp as he prepared to lie out and cure in the cold Alpine winter air.

Fresh Alpine air was not the only form of air considered to be therapeutically useful for consumptive patients. Balzac wrote of a Swiss consumptive who treated himself by inhaling the air from a cow barn. In the 1820s, tuberculosis patients in America were placed in rooms built in barns just above cow stalls, and in 1842 Dr. John Grogan confined his patients to Mammoth Cave, Kentucky to live in darkness illumined only by candles and oil lamps lamps in air redolent from accumulated sewage.[11]

Perhaps the most bizarre measure said to have been employed for strengthening the resistance of tuberculous patients to their disease was the drinking of blood of freshly slaughtered animals. In fact, in 1939, a French newspaper carried a sensationalist report of an eight-year-old boy who was kidnapped in Spain, "gagged and put in a sack. He was then taken to the patient's room, undressed, and then, without being moved by his cries and prayer, the quack plunged his knife into his left axilla. The patient then drank his blood while the boy was dying."[12]

Thomas Sydenham recommended horseback rides for the treatment of tuberculosis in 1742, writing, "the principal assistant in the cure of this disease is riding on horseback every day, insomuch that whoever has recourse to this exercise in order to his cure, need not be tied down to observe any rules in point of diet, nor be debarred any kind of solid or liquid aliment, as the cure depends wholly on exercise."[13] Sydenham was enormously respected in his day, and his medical colleagues immediately accepted and put into practice this recommendation. For many decades, all prescriptions for consumptives included horseback riding. Even as he approached death in Italy in 1820, Keats climbed atop a horse for the gentle rides recommended by Dr. James Clark (Chapter 12).

Sea Voyages were a cornerstone of the treatment of consumptives for centuries. In classic times, Celsus recommended them. Both Keats and Stevenson sought relief on the sea, for by the eighteenth and nineteenth century all experts believed that shipboard life was one of the most effective measures available for the treatment of tuberculosis. At age 21, George Washington accompanied his half-brother Lawrence to Barbados on a voyage seeking recovery from Lawrence's tuberculosis. Not long after his return, Washington was stricken with pleurisy, which as we have seen in the cases of Eleanor Roosevelt and Alice Marble, is sometimes a manifestation of early tuberculosis. There is no evidence that Washington suffered further from tuberculosis, but he was in poor health for about two years following his return from Barbados.

John Warren, one of the founders of Harvard Medical School and himself a sufferer from tuberculosis, strongly advocated sea voyages to Bermuda and the Caribbean. Historian Shiela Rothman elegantly documents the wide acceptance of sea voyages for the treatment of men who, rich or poor, expended their family resources for such expeditions. Women, she points out, were excluded from this form of therapy, for they were expected to continue their duties as wives and mothers in their homes, even in the face of overwhelming illness. Rothman poignantly recounts the story of a New England professor's wife, who was treated by Warren, and her struggles to maintain her home and family while dying of relentlessly progressive tuberculosis.[14]

From wolf's liver to sea voyages, the treatment of tuberculosis evolved over time from magical potions to measures thought to strengthen the bodily resistance of ill patients. Meanwhile, the epidemic of tuberculosis raged. The concept of a therapeutic agent that might cure the disease by specifically attacking its root cause could not emerge until after Koch's demonstration of the causative tubercle bacillus. As we will see, it took nearly seven decades after Koch identified the target in 1882 for such a magic bullet to be found.

20

False Hope

"At this time I conclude only that it is possible to render harmless the pathogenic bacteria that are found in a living body and to do this without disadvantage to the body," stated Robert Koch, the preeminent medical scientist of his time, to an audience of eight thousand physicians on August 3, 1890 at the Tenth International Medical Congress in Berlin.[1] Seldom has there been a more dramatic pronouncement by a more respected authority in the history of medicine. Koch's words launched an immediately accepted form of therapy for the world's most dread disease, a therapy that endured for decades, a therapy that was ultimately discredited. That Koch was badly mistaken was a painful conclusion that the world accepted with remorse. Looking back, one can understand with humility and sympathy that Koch reached his flawed conclusions by reasoning from what seemed at the time an iron-clad data base. Looking forward, one can hope that we today will approach new therapies for dread diseases with minds that are both open and critical, not forgetting that desperation rarely leaves judgement unimpaired.

In Chapter 9 we learned of the life of the extraordinary man Robert Koch; in Chapter 13 of the diagnostic importance of his tuberculin. It is now time to consider the use of tuberculin for the treatment of tuberculosis. The treatment and cure of tuberculosis was, after all, Koch's goal. He was encouraged in his aspirations by the earlier work of Jenner and Pasteur with small pox and rabies and by his own observations on the development of immunity by guinea pigs surviving primary tuberculous infection (Chapter 15). Koch then prepared his tuberculin—the sterilized culture fluid in which tubercle bacilli had been growing—and observed that immune responses in animals could be elicited with this germ-free substance. Was it not logical that the immunity of persons suffering from tuberculosis could be augmented by injections of tuberculin with therapeutic benefit?

Koch began by injecting guinea pigs and then people—himself and other healthy persons—with tuberculin to demonstrate its safety. Healthy guinea pigs tolerated the material without side effects. Koch noted that some healthy persons, including himself, as well as tuberculosis patients developed fever following the injections, thus laying the basis for von Pirquet's development of the tuberculin skin test (Chapter 13). "Three to four hours after the injection", he wrote describing his own reaction to a dose more than twelve thousand times that we now use for tuberculin skin testing, "there came on pain in the limbs, fatigue, inclination to cough, difficulty in breathing, which speedily increased. In the fifth hour an unusually violent attack of ague followed, which lasted almost an hour. At the same time there was sickness, vomiting, and rise of body temperature up to 39.6°C. After twelve hours all these symptoms abated. The temperature fell until next day [sic] it was normal, and a feeling of fatigue and pain in the limbs continued for a few days, and for exactly the same period of time the site of injection remained slightly painful and red."[2] In Koch's judgement such a reaction was tolerable if a therapeutic benefit could be demonstrated. Viewed from the vantage point of current medical knowledge, the reaction that Koch described in himself was probably a combination of delayed hypersensitivity to tuberculin antigens—the reaction recognized by von Pirquet as the basis for a diagnostic skin test—and a reaction to a substance in the cell wall of tubercle bacilli with properties of endotoxin. Endotoxin is a common bacterial component that is responsible for inducing the fever of many infections; it is not present in tubercle bacilli, but related compounds are and seem likely to be the cause of some of the reactions to the enormous amounts of tuberculin Koch used.

Koch's first account of the use of tuberculin for the treatment of tuberculosis was published in the German medical journal *Deutsche Medicinische Wochenschrift* on November 15, 1890. An English translation appeared in the *British Medical Journal* one week later, and *The Lancet*, a prominent British medical journal published a precis of Koch's paper on the same date.[3] After describing his demonstration of the safety of tuberculin, he described its use in patients with lupus vulgaris, tuberculosis of the skin. The response to treatment was easily observed in such patients. A series of weekly injections were given, continuing until the reaction to the injections weakened and ceased. "In two cases of facial lupus," Koch reported, "the lupus spots were thus brought to complete cicatrization [scarring—TMD] by three or four injections; the other lupus cases improved in proportion to the duration of treatment. All these patients had been sufferers for many years, having been previously treated unsuccessfully by various therapeutic methods."[4] Koch then noted that he had similarly treated cases of glandular, bone, and joint tuberculosis. "The result was the same as in the lupus cases—a speedy cure in recent and slight cases, slow improvement in severe cases."

With respect to pulmonary tuberculosis—"phthisical cases" in Koch's words—Koch was more cautious. He noted that they tolerated tuberculin injections poorly, and for this reason he was forced to use low doses. He also noted that the response of these patients was less easy to observe directly than that of those patients with more superficial forms of disease. None-the-less, Koch reported improvement in the symptoms of patients in the early stages of disease and concluded that "phthisis in the beginning can be cured with certainty by this remedy." Advanced cases, he postulated, might be benefitted for a time but would "only obtain lasting benefit from the remedy in exceptional cases."

In a telling statement that concluded his report, Koch said, "Finally I would remark that I have purposely omitted statistical accounts and descriptions of individual cases, because the medical men who furnished us with patients for our investigations have themselves decided to publish the description of their cases, and I wished my account to be as objective as possible, leaving to them all that is purely personal." Even in Koch's day, when scientific investigations were conducted with less scrutiny than they are today, that statement is remarkable. It suggests that Koch, convinced as he was of the benefit of tuberculin, was less than objective in gathering his clinical data. It may reveal a tragic lapse in the work of one of history's most brilliant and most rigorous medical scientists.

From a modern perspective, we can understand what Koch observed and what he and his contemporaries believed to be therapeutic benefit from injections of tuberculin. First of all, Koch observed what is now known as the focal response. When large doses of the antigens in tuberculin are given, there is an allergic flare-up of the tissue response at the site of disease. This flare-up may lead to scarring, and in this manner the small skin lesions of lupus vulgaris may be obliterated. The more extensive lesions of tuberculosis in its usual sites in lungs are not significantly altered by these focal responses. Secondly, Koch observed a combination of desensitization to tuberculin antigens and tolerance to endotoxin. Desensitization is the phenomenon that occurs when an offending antigen is injected repeatedly into an allergic subject. Desensitization is widely used today in the treatment of allergies. Today's allergists, however, use doses carefully designed to be too small to elicit major reactions. Tolerance to endotoxin occurs when bacterial products are given repeatedly. Patients with severe infections may have less and less fever with each succeeding wave of blood-born bacteria. Thus, possibly for a combination of reasons, Koch observed that with repeated injections, his patients suffered fewer and fewer symptoms from the tuberculin itself.

Tuberculin therapy for tuberculosis was accepted by physicians and patients with a rapidity unparalleled in medical history. Koch and his colleagues immediately began producing tuberculin for others, and within days of Koch's presentation in Berlin his assistants began holding demonstrations of its use.[5] The *British Medical Journal*'s translation of Koch's paper is immediately followed by an account of a series of reports of patients treated in Berlin with tuberculin and described or demonstrated to an eager audience of physicians at the same conference at which Koch spoke. While some improvement was described, these reports were all more cautious than was Koch.[6]

Doctors and patients alike flocked to Berlin. Leading hospitals sent delegations. Koch and his colleagues produced tuberculin and supplied it to physicians, although they kept its composition secret. With a year, this therapy had been administered to several thousand patients. Paul Erlich, the eminent chemist who had heard Koch's original description of the tubercle bacillus and then developed substantial improvements in the staining technique used to identify these organisms (Chapter 9), made his own diagnosis of tuberculosis by finding the bacilli in his sputum. He became a patient, and he was among the early recipients of injections of tuberculin for the treatment of tuberculosis.

Arthur Conan Doyle, the author of the Sherlock Holmes mystery stories, was a respected London physician. His wife had tuberculosis.

He was one of the first British physicians to travel to Berlin to learn Koch's method of tuberculin therapy. He had remarkable insight into the effects of tuberculin injections, and he pointed out that Koch's lymph did nothing to attack the tubercle bacillus itself. Rather, he believed, it led to the destruction of tissues harboring tubercle bacilli, causing their expulsion from the body. Only rarely, Doyle felt, would this expulsion be so complete as to remove totally the pathogenic bacteria.[7] Drs. Flick and Trudeau, pioneers in the treatment of tuberculosis in the United States about whom we will learn more in the next chapter, obtained samples of Koch's tuberculin and tried it on their patients.

A circus atmosphere developed around tuberculin therapy. Koch's colleagues conducted public demonstrations at which patients were injected with tuberculin. In a widely circulated essay, Arthur Conan Doyle likened Europe's response to Koch's announcement to that of people in the middle ages to a religious miracle or the establishment of a new "wonder-working shrine." The cover of the issue of the London periodical containing Doyle's essay represented Koch as St. George slaying a dragon tubercle bacillus.[8] The Prussian government prepared to build a special hospital devoted to Koch's treatment.

The British journal, *The Lancet*, was at that time and remains today a major forum for the communication of new medical information and the exchange of ideas relating to medical practice. Beginning with the publication of its precis of Koch's report on November 22, 1890, the Lancet's pages were filled with reports and divergent opinions concerning Koch's remedy. An editorial accompanying the first report set the stage by expressing caution about the potential for cure with tuberculin therapy.[9] In an earlier editorial, however, the editors of Lancet had been unrestrained in their excitement over Koch's work. "Indeed," they concluded "apart from the fact that we may be on the verge of a revolution in therapeutics, it may be said that bacteriology itself is on its trial in this momentous investigation."[10] However, on December 20, 1890, a scathing letter to the editors of Lancet derided the publicity by which, "day after day the gaping multitude were informed how 'Dr. This' or 'Dr. That' having received a sample of the precious fluid had proceeded to inject it in the presence of a circle of admiring and envious *confrères*. The ceremonial. . . . might have been the performance of a sacred rite."[11] On the same date, another correspondent wrote, "This is a most hysterical age. But why should men of science lose their heads and follow in the hue-and-cry of the unreasoning multitude?"[12] On the other hand, a special correspondent from Berlin, writing in the same issue of Lancet and commenting on the autopsy findings of a patient reported to have died as a result of Koch's tuberculin therapy, sought to allay fears that Koch's remedy might actually have caused the patient's demise.[13]

The denouement came in April 1891, less than a year after Koch's original claim of therapeutic efficacy for tuberculin. A Prussian government commission headed by Professor Guttstadt, a statistician, reported on the results of the treatment of two thousand, one hundred and seventy-two patients treated with a total of nearly eighteen thousand injections of tuberculin. Fewer than one in five were considered substantially improved, and most of them were cases of lupus vulgaris. The toxicity of treatment was great, and over-all more patients died than improved during treatment. While it could not be concluded that tuberculin was causing the deaths in these desperately ill persons, it was abundantly evident that tuberculin therapy was accompanied by severe side reactions and that its benefit was marginal for most patients.[14]

Tuberculin did not die easily, for the hope for a magic bullet capable of curing tuberculosis resonated in the hearts and minds of many patients and the physicians who cared for them. In 1948, more than a half century after the bright hope of tuberculin had been extinguished in the minds of most experts, the distinguished tuberculosis physician Francis Marion Pottenger, devoted a chapter in his text on tuberculosis to tuberculin therapy. Pottenger clearly understood the need to desensitize patients to tuberculin, and for this purpose he embraced the use of very small initial doses with progressive increases in subsequent doses. By this method, he avoided severe reactions, just as modern allergists avoid severe reactions in desensitizing allergic patients. "Can the administration of tuberculin aid the patient to an extent beyond that of the natural infection in building up a specific defense?" Pottenger asked. His reply was strongly affirmative.[15]

Tuberculin therapy and Pottenger's text are both unknown in medical practice today. Tuberculosis is cured by effective chemotherapeutic drugs. The only use of tuberculin is for diagnosis. But Koch was correct in thinking that a patient's immune responses have a primary role in defense against tuberculous infection. For his time, his thinking was clear and his hypotheses supportable. Where he and almost the entire medical community of his day went astray was in letting hope, compassion, and desire outpace science and reason. Medicine is an art; medicine is also a science.

21

Places Apart

Thomas Mann was thirty-seven years old in 1912. He had already been acclaimed for his novel *Buddenbrooks*, the major work cited when he received the Nobel Prize for literature in 1929. In 1912, he went to Davos, Switzerland to visit his ailing tuberculous wife. Like Hans Castorp, the hero of his later classic *The Magic Mountain*, Mann took advantage of his visit to the famous center for chest diseases to be examined by a leading specialist, and like his hero, Mann learned in that way that he suffered from tuberculosis.[1] Mann refused the recommended retreat to convalescence in the famous Alpine spa, but he built his later novel on his brief experience there. *The Magic Mountain* offered a metaphorical and critical view of life in the flat land below from the isolated, other-worldly vantage point offered by both the disease tuberculosis and the remote place in which it was treated.

The removal of consumptive patients to places apart may have been justified later for its role in limiting the spread of tuberculous infection, but the practice began in Germany before tuberculosis was generally considered to be contagious. Herman Brehmer was a young physician practicing in the village of Goerbersdorf in Prussia. He had developed an interest in tuberculosis while studying as a medical student, and his required degree thesis discussed his views of the cause of this disease. He attributed tuberculosis to an abnormal ratio in the size of the lungs and the heart, and he concluded that high altitudes would ameliorate consumption by acting to correct this size disparity. The Silesian Mountains locale of Goerbersdof, he felt, was ideal for treating persons with tuberculosis, and in 1859 he opened what is generally considered to be the first sanatorium devoted to the treatment of tuberculosis. Brehmer's Heilanstalt became famous, and its program of rest, a rich diet, and supervised exercise was widely copied.[2] Brehmer's assistant and pupil,

Peter Detweiler, opened a similar sanatorium in Falkenstien, near Frankfort, in 1867.

The mile high valley of Davos in Eastern Switzerland became reputed as a place favorable for the treatment of scrofula in the early 1840s, and by the mid 1860s patients with pulmonary tuberculosis were flocking to its many hostels and sanatoria catering to consumptive patients. Arthur Conan Doyle brought his tuberculous wife there in the 1860s. As we have noted, Robert Louis Stevenson sought treatment there two decades later. Today, Davos is one of the premier ski resorts of Europe; its sanatoria have been replaced by luxury tourist hotels.

The first facility devoted to the care of patients with tuberculosis established in North America was the Channing Home opened in the basement of a Boston church in May 1857, two years before Brehmer opened his Heilanstalt in Silesia. Its site was determined by opportunity, not consideration of physiologic theories, and there is no more poignant story in medical history than that of Harriet Ryan Albee, the founder of the Channing Home.[3] Harriet Ryan was born in Boston in 1829. Her father was disabled by an explosion in the quarry where he worked, and Harriet's mother Elizabeth Cannon Ryan became the mainstay of the family and a role model for her daughter. Elizabeth was a religious woman, and she spent hours in the care of sick and dying women without compensation, doing what she considered God's work and setting a model of service to others for her daughter.

The Ryan family was soon touched by tuberculosis. One of Harriet's sisters died of the disease. Her brother fell ill with it, and then Harriet herself contracted tuberculosis. But consumption was not a reason for women to fall behind in their work, and Harriet found employment as a lady's maid, a dressmaker, and then a hair dresser. At night, following in her mother's footsteps, Harriet devoted herself to the care of sick women, many of whom had tuberculosis. In 1857 she persuaded the minister of the Federal Street Church located on Channing Street to lease her the church basement for one hundred dollars a month. She brought sick and dying tuberculous women to the church, providing much of the nursing care for them herself and obtaining food for them by standing in line at a pauper's soup kitchen. During the next two years, fifty-two patients were admitted, of whom eighteen died.

Harriet Ryan's efforts attracted the attention of prominent Bostonians, and soon money became available to support her home. Ralph Waldo Emerson, who suffered from tuberculosis himself, James Russell Lowell, and Oliver Wendell Holmes all became supporters. The home moved to larger quarters, and became a well endowed and recognized institution for the treatment of tuberculosis. Ultimately, in 1907, the Channing Home moved into a substantial building on Pilgrim Road opposite the New England Deaconess Hospital. In that location it continued to treat tuberculosis patients for the next fifty years. When it closed in 1958, its endowment funds were transferred to the Harvard Medical School to support the Channing Research Laboratory for the study of infectious diseases.

Harriet Ryan married John Albee in 1864, seven years after the founding of the Channing Home. Her life as wife and mother was a happy one, but her tuberculosis progressed and she became increasingly ill. A sea voyage to the Bahamas did not help her. Finally, she herself became a patient at the Channing Home, where she died on May 2, 1873 at the age of forty-four, sixteen years after she brought her first patient to the church basement on Channing Street. In 1987 the Harvard Medical School established the Harriet Ryan Albee Professorship of Medicine to honor this courageous woman.

In February 1873 Edward Livingston Trudeau, a man destined to have an effect on medical practice in the treatment of tuberculosis unparalleled even by Koch, presented himself for an examination at the office of Dr. Edward Janeway, one of New York City's most eminent diagnosticians, because of fever that had failed to respond to treatment for malaria with quinine. "Well, Dr. Janeway, you can find nothing the matter?" asked the young physician Trudeau. "Yes," came the reply, "the upper two-thirds of the left lung is involved in an active tuberculous process." Trudeau was stunned, for he knew tuberculosis well. In his words, "It seemed to me the world had suddenly grown dark. The sun was shining, it is true, and the street was filled with the rush and noise of traffic, but to me the world had lost every vestige of brightness. I had consumption—that most fatal of diseases! . . . It meant death and I had never thought of death before! Was I ready to die? How could I tell my wife?"[4]

Edward Livingston Trudeau was born in New York on October 5, 1848 into a world of affluence, the descendent of several generations of physicians.[5] He grew up in Paris, living with his mother, who had separated from his father. At the age of seventeen he returned to New York and, despite the problems of conquering a nearly unknown language, soon entered into the social whirl of well-to-do young people of that metropolis. With little real sense of vocation, he decided to become a naval officer. He entered a military preparatory school at Newport, and an influential friend secured an appointment for him at the United States Naval Academy. But he was not destined to become a naval officer.

Trudeau's brother, Francis, to whom he was very close, developed active tuberculosis in September 1865, only a few months after Trudeau's return to the United States. Plans for a naval education were put aside, and Trudeau devoted himself to the care of his brother, sharing his bedroom, nursing him, and caring for him as he approached his death in December. One cannot but be struck by the parallel with the bedside devotion of John Keats to his mother and later his brother during their terminal consumptive illnesses.

Trudeau moved to New York City. His life was one of leisure, often focused on the Union Club, with little evident direction or purpose. More or less by default or in accedence to the medical traditions of his heritage, he entered the Columbia University College of Physicians and Surgeons in 1868. He was not a distinguished medical student. Looking back after a long and noteworthy career, Trudeau noted that "the requirements for a medical student in those days were of the simplest." Tuberculosis was taught by the respected but intimidating Dr. Alonzo Clark who, in those years preceding Koch's work, considered it a non-contagious, inherited disease. When one of Trudeau's classmates became ill with tuberculosis, Dr. Clark advised Trudeau, "Tell your friend to go to the mountains and become a stage driver for a few years." Perhaps Trudeau recalled these words when he faced his own diagnosis of tuberculosis a few years later.

Trudeau was in love with Lottie Beare, whom he had met shortly after arriving in the United States. During his student years, he visited her frequently. In 1871, shortly after his medical school commencement, he and Lottie were married. A trip to Europe, a desultory rural practice on Long Island, and the birth of their first child marked the ensuing year. The couple was not pressed for money—both had incomes from family inheritances—but Trudeau found the country life lacking in challenge. The couple moved to New York City, where

Dr. Fessenden Otis, one of Trudeau's medical school professors, offered him a partnership. A second child arrived. Trudeau was happy and felt fulfilled both professionally and personally.

Within two years the Captain of Death had begun its long, stalking pursuit of Trudeau. Having been given his fateful diagnosis, Trudeau tried to reorder his life to accommodate his illness. As recommended by Dr. Janeway, he began a regimen of daily horseback rides. But he worsened, with more fever. He became unable to work. Recalling a happy trip to the Adirondacks two years earlier, he set out on the three day journey to Paul Smith's Adirondack hunting lodge in the company of his good friend Lou Livingston in May 1873. His wife and the two small children went to her parents' home in Little Neck on Long Island. The trip north was arduous. Trudeau was met by Paul Smith, who picked him up and carried him to his bed saying, "Why, Doctor, you don't weigh no more than a dried lamb-skin!" Thus began Trudeau's life in the Adirondacks, a life that would span more than four further decades and that would have an enormous impact on the treatment of tuberculosis.

Trudeau's health slowly improved. He enjoyed the outdoor ambiance, hunting and fishing. Indeed, on his first day he shot a deer from a litter rigged on a boat. Later in the summer he was joined by the wealthy railroad entrepreneur, E. H. Harriman, and Trudeau's Adirondack life became one of outdoor sportsmanship in the company of good friends and optimistic enthusiasts for life in the Adirondacks. In September, Trudeau felt well enough to return to his family.

During the next few years, Trudeau abandoned medicine, devoting much of his life to the rugged wilderness life of the Adirondacks. In 1875 Lottie and the children joined him, and they spent that winter at Paul Smith's. In Trudeau's words, "Up to 1880 I did little but hunt and fish. . . ." However, Trudeau's physician friends were beginning to send tuberculous patients to the Adirondacks to partake of the healthy air that was so benefitting him. Trudeau was aware of the work of Brehmer and Detweiler and their German sanatoria, and the idea of building a sanatorium for consumptives in the Adirondacks began to grow in his mind. He found a suitable site in Saranac Lake, and in 1884, with a gift of twenty-five hundred dollars from D. Willis James, he opened the Adirondack Cottage Sanitarium. Trudeau was a good money raiser with many wealthy friends, and within a few years his sanatorium had grown

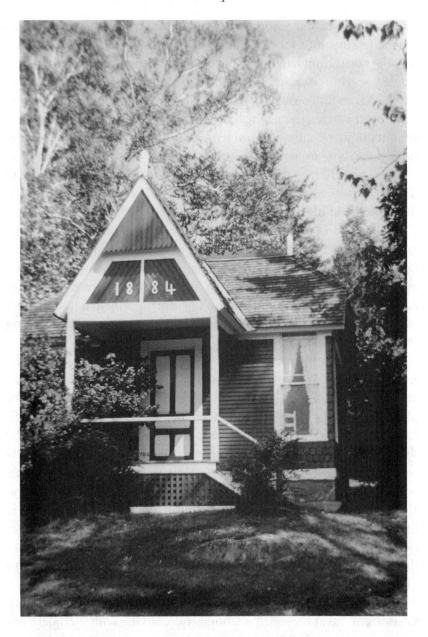

Figure 21.1 Little Red, a restored cottage from Edward Livingston Trudeau's Cottage Sanatorium at Saranac Lake, New York opened in 1884. Little Red was considerably more substantial than the cottages used by most tuberculosis sanatoria of that time. Photograph by the author.

and become one of the world's best known and most successful facilities for the treatment of tuberculous patients. Two decades after its founding, the sanatorium had thirty-six buildings on sixty acres of grounds. It housed one hundred and fifty patients. The town of Saranac Lake became a haven for consumptives. Other cottages were built, and the balconies and porches upon which the victims of tuberculosis rested in the mountain air became a prominent local architectural feature. Other physicians came to Saranac Lake, and joined Trudeau in making daily rounds to minister to the ill. Among them, Dr. Edwin Baldwin came to Trudeau, first as a patient, then as a colleague and collaborator, both in his clinical and his research activities.

While Robert Louis Stevenson was destined to become Trudeau's most famous patient, he was not the only prominent person to seek good health at Saranac Lake. Many among Trudeau's patients were physicians, and many of them returned to the communities from which they came and went on to apply Trudeau's treatment principles to other patients and disseminate the knowledge of this disease that was mounting in the Adirondacks.

Trudeau's treatment regimen of rest, outdoor air, and a hearty diet might have made his sanatorium popular among the patients who cured at Saranac Lake, but it alone would not have secured Trudeau his major place in the history of American medicine. Trudeau, a desultory medical student and a dilettante physician, developed during his years in the Adirondacks into a true medical scientist whose work won him early recognition. He had had little or no training in investigative medicine, and he lived at the time when such European giants as Pasteur and Koch were just elucidating the infectious nature of many diseases. He lived and worked in an isolated site where obtaining any medical reports was difficult. Yet Trudeau seemed to have an inborn ability to design elegant experiments and an unquenchable thirst for knowledge of the disease that continued to plague him.

Trudeau read Koch's papers, and in the same year that he opened his sanatorium, he also opened a laboratory. Working with a crudely improvised incubator in 1885, he became the first person in North America to cultivate the tubercle bacillus. He obtained a microscope and went to New York to learn the technique of staining tubercle bacilli in sputum from Dr. T. Mitchell Prudden, who had studied with Koch. This

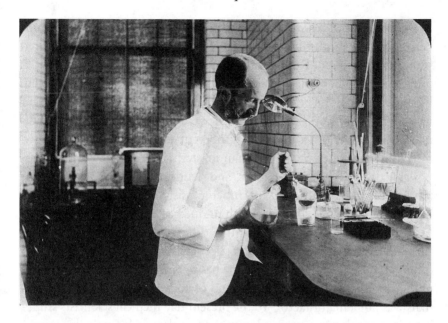

Figure 21.2. Edward Livingston Trudeau in his laboratory at Saranac lake in 1895. Photograph courtesy of the American Lung Association.

proved to be a daunting task, but Trudeau persisted at it until he mastered the technique. Later, when Trudeau's laboratory was destroyed by fire, Prudden sent a gift to Trudeau of a replacement instrument.

Trudeau chose rabbits as experimental animals, and he almost instinctively designed carefully controlled experiments that were immediately accepted by his medical peers. He infected rabbits, allowing some the free run of an island and confining others in close and dark quarters. The free-roaming rabbits remained healthy; the confined animals became diseased. Like Koch, Trudeau was interested in immunity to tuberculosis. Using materials from his cultures and working independently and with only limited knowledge of Koch's studies, Trudeau failed to demonstrate immunity in rabbits from injections of materials very similar to the tuberculin used by Koch. Whole, living organisms were required to establish immunity. Additionally, Trudeau observed that strains of tubercle bacilli passed serially in culture lost much of their virulence, presaging the vaccine development work of Calmette and Guérin (Chapter 15).[6]

In his report of his studies, Trudeau very clearly summarized his understanding of immunity to tuberculosis, both native and that acquired from prior infection. Read today, Trudeau's ideas have ring of truth that provokes awe when one considers the time in which they were written. How different the next few years of the history of tuberculosis might have been if his experiments, which were published almost simultaneously with Koch's descriptions of tuberculin therapy, had been heeded instead of the words of the German master!

Why did two scientists, Koch and Trudeau, obtain such different results in their experiments with tuberculosis? One cannot be sure. Perhaps Koch interpreted his data with undue haste, but individual strains of rabbits and guinea pigs react quite differently to tuberculous infection, and different strains of tubercle bacilli are variously virulent in different animal study systems. One has to wonder if the happenstance of the choices of strain of bacteria and of convenient experimental animals was not a major factor. To the present day medical scientists studying tuberculosis must contend with the fact that each particular experimental system used for experiments is sufficiently distinct so that it is often difficult to generalize from experimental results, no matter how carefully the research is done.

Trudeau's peers recognized him, respected him, and bestowed many honors upon him. Yale, Pennsylvania, McGill, and Columbia Universities all awarded him honorary degrees. Towards the end of his life he refused other degrees and awards, as he was too ill to travel to accept them. He was elected president of the American Congress of Physicians and Surgeons. His tuberculosis treatment regimen was described and recommended by Sir William Osler in his classic and pioneering medical textbook.

Trudeau was a founding member and the first president in 1904 of the National Association for the Study and Prevention of Tuberculosis, now the American Lung Association, a major voluntary health organization promoting lung health. The American Sanatorium Association was founded a year later to provide a scientific forum for physicians caring for patients in tuberculosis sanatoria; in 1939, it was renamed the American Trudeau Society in his honor. Today, as the American Thoracic Society, it remains a major professional society for pulmonary physicians.

More than four decades passed as Trudeau made his rounds among the many patients who joined him at Saranac Lake and as he himself and his family suffered from the ravages of that disease. He was frequently ill. In 1893, his daughter Chatte died of tuberculosis. A decade later his son Ned, who had followed Trudeau into medicine, died. In his autobiography, Trudeau attributed Ned's death to a blood clot in the lungs (pulmonary embolus) following an episode of pneumonia. In 1906 Trudeau's health began to fail once more, progressively and relentlessly. Near the end, a left pneumothorax (Chapter 22) brought no improvement. He died quietly at his home in Saranac Lake on November 15, 1915, a victim of the disease to which he had devoted his energies throughout his singularly productive life.

Trudeau's laboratory rose from its humble beginnings to become a leader in tuberculosis research. Under the directorship of William Steenken, it carried out many pioneering microbiological studies that paved the way for trials of many new drugs for the treatment of tuberculosis. In 1954, when the now well-endowed Adirondack Cottage Sanitarium faced closing, obsolete in the time of drug treatment of tuberculosis, the trustees used its resources to open and endow a new laboratory on the grounds of the sanatorium, naming it the Trudeau Institute. Trudeau's grandson, Francis B. Trudeau, a physician who practiced in Saranac Lake, was the first to chair the board of the new institute. A life-sized bronze statue by Gutzon Borlum of Edward Livingston Trudeau, reclining on a chaise and wrapped in robes of the sort used by his patients, graces the lawn. At the base of the statue are carved the memorable words, "Guérir quelquefois, soulanger souvent, consoler toujours." To cure sometimes, to relieve often, to comfort always. To Trudeau, this call was to both the physician and the scientist.

In the spring of 1881, just a year before Koch's dramatic description of the tubercle bacillus and eight years after Trudeau's desperate journey to the Adirondack shelter of Paul Smith's lodge, Dr. Lawrence F. Flick, a young physician in Philadelphia, learned that he had tuberculosis. A trip west failed to improve his health. As he struggled against the burden of his illness to establish himself as a physician, he became increasingly concerned about both the plight of his fellow sufferers and the spread of tuberculosis in the community. He believed tuberculosis to be contagious, a view still not shared by most of his medical colleagues,

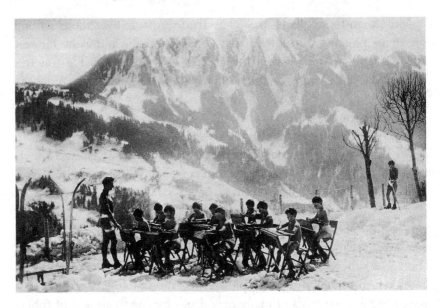

Figure 21.3. Children dressed only in undershorts in an outdoor school class at Dr. Rollier's Institute for Heliotherapy Treatment in Leysin, Switzerland. Photograph courtesy of the American Lung Association.

and he argued with increasing stridor that the government ought to shoulder the burden of isolating as a public health measure and caring for as a humanitarian act those poor consumptives who could not afford private hospital care.[7]

Flick's stridor gave way to action. Increasingly his medical practice was devoted to the care of patients with tuberculosis, many of whom were poor or destitute. Both Catholic and Episcopal churches in Philadelphia provided shelter for homeless tuberculosis victims, and Flick brought his healing art to those whom the churches sheltered. In 1895, he organized the Pennsylvania Society for the Prevention of Tuberculosis, the first such patient advocacy organization and the progenitor of modern Christmas Seal organizations. In the same year, with the assistance of two Catholic sodalities, he organized the Free Hospital for Poor Consumptives. Lacking a physical facility, the Free Hospital strove to care for its patients in a variety of medical settings where it paid for their accommodations.

Flick wanted to establish a mountain sanatorium similar to that of Trudeau for his Free Hospital's penniless patients. Elwell Stockdale, one of Flick's affluent patients, led the way. Stockdale had cured in a variety of well known locations in Europe and North America and finally retreated to a farm house in White Haven on the banks of the Lehigh River in Northeastern Pennsylvania. Stockdale offered his barn as a camp for Flick's impoverished patients. Rudimentary living accommodations were constructed in the barn, and in August 1901 the first three tuberculous patients took up residence there.

Life at White Haven was Spartan, and it was probably typical of that in many early tuberculosis sanatoria. Fresh air, rest, and regulated exercise were the bulwarks of the treatment regimen. Comfort was not viewed as salutary. The winter was cold in the unheated barn, and the patients shivered beneath the few available blankets. Flick was particularly concerned with the diet of his patients; a report from Stockdale noted that, "one man had seventeen glasses of milk and eight raw eggs yesterday and another fourteen and eight."[8]

The White Haven Sanatorium attracted attention in Philadelphia. Philanthropic donations arrived, and the facility expanded. By 1906 the sanatorium had grown to house one hundred and seventy-two patients in its cottages, and central administration and kitchen facilities had been constructed. Nurses were employed, as were resident physicians, most of whom were recent medical school graduates suffering from tuberculosis themselves. Medical care was supervised by physicians living in the community of White Haven. In that year, Flick hired Dr. G. Justice Ewing as a full time medical director. This action marked a fundamental change at White Haven and mirrored a general change in sanatoria in the prevailing approach to medical care in tuberculosis facilities. Whether in Saranac Lake, Davos, or White Haven, sanatoria of the day provided shelter, while medical care was provided by local practitioners. In some cases, as with Trudeau in Saranac Lake, the local physician might also be the proprietor of the sanatorium, but more often than not this was not the case. Dr. Ewing assumed responsibility for all of the patients at White Haven, and the sanatorium became a true hospital rather than a rest home. A new pattern for the care of patients with tuberculosis was thus established and with it a new and more institutionalized approach to the disease itself. However, money

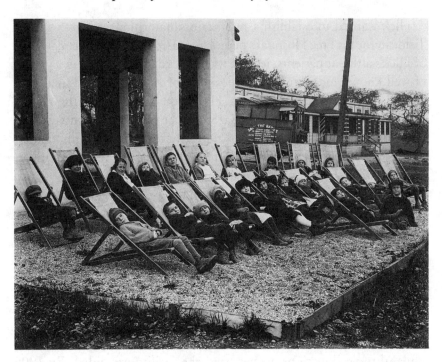

Figure 21.4. Children partaking of rest and fresh air at Sunny Acres Sanatorium in Cuyahoga County, Ohio, April 6, 1918. Rest in the open air was a regular feature of sanatorium life. Naming one of its two tuberculosis hospitals "Sunny Acres" was an ironic act for Cuyahoga County, for this hospital sat near the highest point in the county in what local residents call "the snow belt," where lake effect snow produced by wind across Lake Erie creates the most awesome winter weather of the region. Photograph courtesy of the American Lung Association of Northern Ohio.

to pay Ewing soon was lacking, and White Haven reverted to its prior system of local physicians and residents who staffed the hospital in return for free care for their tuberculosis. Ewing, who also suffered from the disease, was told he could practice in the community and charge his patients at White Haven. He declined this arrangement and moved with his wife to Lunenberg, Massachusetts, where he opened his own tuberculosis treatment facility but succumbed three years later to his illness.[9]

Flick's interest in tuberculosis, like that of Trudeau, extended beyond

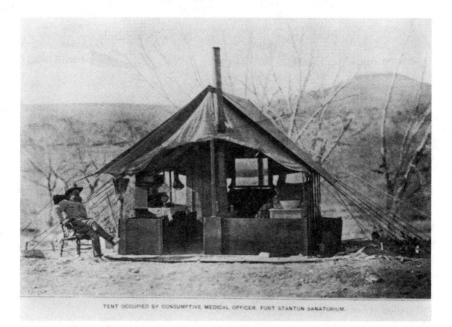

Figure 21.5. Tent occupied by a tuberculous medical officer at the Fort Stanton Sanatorium in New Mexico. Photograph courtesy of the American Lung Association.

the care of those ill with this disease. In 1903, with a gift from Henry Phipps, Flick opened the Henry Phipps Institute for the Study, Prevention, and Treatment of Tuberculosis in Philadelphia. Later to become a unit of the University of Pennsylvania, this institute differed from other facilities for the study of tuberculosis in that it sought to combine patient care with research. Many distinguished scientists made it home, including Max Lurie (Chapter 14), Esmond R. Long, Florence Seibert (Chapter 13), and Joseph Aronson (Chapter 15). The leaders of American medicine in the sanatorium era, Trudeau and Flick among them, recognized that solving the problem presented by the tuberculosis epidemic they faced required more than good patient care. It required better understanding of the disease. It required new modalities of prevention and cure. It required a vigorous biomedical research program.

Plagued not only by his tuberculosis but also by diabetes, Flick approached his elder years in chronic ill health, confined to his home,

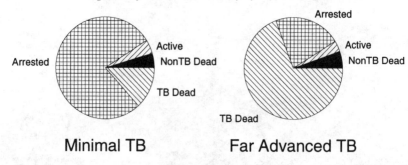

Minimal TB   ## Far Advanced TB

Figure 21.6. Status at fifteen years after admission of patients hospitalized in New York State sanatoria with minimal and far advanced tuberculosis. Of those with minimal tuberculosis at admission, the majority were classified as arrested fifteen years later. Of those with far advanced disease, the majority had died of their disease. Overall, the tuberculosis mortality was thirty-nine percent. Data from Alling DW, Bosworth ER. The after history of pulmonary tuberculosis. VI. The first fifteen years following diagnosis. Am Rev Respir Dis 1960; 81:839-849.

often bed-ridden. He died on July 7, 1938 in the central Philadelphia home where he had lived and practiced medicine during an extraordinary life devoted to the care of consumptives and to leadership in efforts to mount and win a campaign against this captain of death.

The sanatoria founded by Herman Brehmer, Harriet Ryan, Edward Trudeau, and Lawrence Flick were pace setters. Other similar institutions followed quickly. Indeed, by 1904 there were one hundred and fifteen tuberculosis treatment facilities in the United States with approximately eight thousand beds. By 1923, the number had grown to six hundred and fifty-six, with more than sixty-six thousand beds; by 1953, eight hundred and thirty-nine sanatoria with more than one hundred and thirty-thousand beds.[10] The average cost of hospitalization at that time was approximately fifteen dollars per day, so that in the United States nearly one million dollars was being spent each day on hospital care for tuberculosis patients as the country entered the second half of the twentieth century and the era of drug treatment for this disease.[11]

Life in a tuberculosis sanatorium was an other-world experience. Entire social structures developed within these institutions, focused on rituals related to the disease. Thomas Mann captured this element of sanatorium life in rich detail in his account of Hans Castorp's life at Davos.[12] Once ill and once determined to seek cure in a sanatorium, one entered its world apart without knowledge of what the outcome might be. The patient surrendered control of life and being to the sanatorium and its demigod doctors. In the words of Hofrat Behrens, Mann's Magic Mountain physician, one "doesn't get well from one day to the next."[13] This was the indefinite sentence imposed by the judge of the high court from which there was no appeal. How then could a patient be concerned with the world left behind? How then could a patient do other than surrender to the institution and its peculiarly encapsulated society?

Not all of the places apart in which those afflicted with tuberculosis sought cure were in Davos, Saranac Lake, or White Haven. Many were more rugged and even more remote. Camping, hunting, and living a primitive out-of-doors life of privation in the American West became an accepted mode of treatment.[14] The building of railroads during the latter half of the nineteenth century opened the West further to ailing Americans. One could reach the land of health and happiness more easily, and land speculators aggressively promoted some locales as healing centers. Retired General William Jackson Palmer touted his development of Colorado Springs on the basis of its salubrious setting, having lured a railroad company into building a spur line to the new community. California was another favored site for curing. Pasadena was founded as a center for the cure of consumption; decades later, Alice Marble was hospitalized at the Pottenger Sanatorium in Monrovia, only ten miles east of Pasadena (Chapter 18). Robert Louis Stevenson, it will be recalled, camped out in California in the vicinity of Monterrey (Chapter 12).

How effective was sanatorium treatment for tuberculosis? What happened to patients who entered those places? Were they cured? Or did they remain ill and die of their disease? Those questions were addressed in 1960 by David Alling, who himself had been a tuberculosis patient in a sanatorium and honed his interest in statistics during his confinement, and Edward Bosworth.[15] They reviewed the records of five hundred and sixty-four persons who were hospitalized in sanatoria New York State during the decade 1938 to 1948. Their review encompassed fifteen years after admission to a tuberculosis facility. The major determinant of outcome proved to be the extent of disease at the time of hospitalization. Twenty-three percent had disease classified as minimal.[16] The tuberculosis of seventy percent of these minimally diseased patients was considered arrested by five years after hospitalization, and this favorable outcome continued, with seventy-eight percent inactive at fifteen years. Thirteen percent of these individuals had died of tuberculosis at the time of the fifteen year review.

The outlook was less favorable for patients with more extensive disease. Among thirty-seven percent of patients who were admitted with disease considered moderately advanced, the tuberculosis was considered arrested in fifty-eight percent after five years. However, further relapses occurred, and only fifty-five percent were considered arrested after fifteen years. Twenty-three percent of these persons had died of tuberculosis at the fifteen year follow-up time. Forty-one percent of the patients were judged to have far advanced disease at the time of hospitalization, and their outlook was grim, indeed. Half died within the first two years, and after five years, sixty percent were dead of tuberculosis. Only twenty-two percent achieved the desired goal of arrested disease. Figure 21.6 contrasts the outlook for patients treated in sanatoria who entered with either minimal or far advanced disease. For those with far advanced tuberculosis, the prognosis was dismal, indeed—worse, in fact, than for most forms of cancer today. Despite the enormous effort expended in the care of its victims during the sanatorium era, tuberculosis remained a captain of death.

Collapse and Mutilation

As Edward Livingston Trudeau approached the end of his life, his health continuing to fail before the relentless destruction of his lungs by tuberculosis, he decided to submit to the induction of a pneumothorax, a procedure intended to collapse his left lung. Surely, such a draconian measure could not be expected to help the dying physician who already suffered from shortness of breath. In fact, it did not benefit Trudeau,[1] and in retrospect it probably increased his symptoms and may have hastened his demise. It certainly left him with less functioning lung to support his already diminished respiratory capacity, and it probably forced his weakened heart to pump blood through pulmonary blood vessels futilely in a quest for oxygen no longer there. The induction of a pneumothorax was still an unproven treatment at that time. Its efficacy was uncertain, and its safety was a matter of continuing debate. Pneumothorax had to that date only rarely been used at Trudeau's sanatorium. Why then did the man who understood tuberculosis far better than almost any other person of his time accept this form of therapy? Trudeau may have acted out of desperation, but there were precedents and an established rationale for the use of pneumothorax for tuberculosis. Moreover, the same thinking that led to the use of this procedure ultimately resulted in the adoption of even more radical measures to collapse tuberculous lungs.

Dettweiler in Europe and Trudeau in North America introduced bed rest into the management of tuberculosis at their sanatoria. Treatment regimens varied a great deal in tuberculosis sanatoria, but rest increasingly became a central part of the routine in most of these institutions. Even in the bitter winter, lying out on open porches was thought to be of great benefit.[2] Sand bags were sometimes used to hold a patient's body in place, interdicting unnecessary movement, and patients were not allowed to put their hands behind their head for fear of stretching the lungs. The idea that resting a diseased lung as completely as possible would lead to the healing of pulmonary tuberculosis was an extension of the belief in the value of bed rest. Since even bed-bound patients still must move their lungs in breathing, would it not be of benefit to patients if diseased portions of lung could be made motionless? It was further thought that compression of lung tissue would bring inflamed surfaces into opposition and promote healing and scarring in the same fashion that a wound heals when its edges are brought together. Areas of disease with cavities were expected to benefit especially from such management.

The lungs lie within the chest and are expanded passively by the muscles of the chest wall and the diaphragm, the great dome-shaped muscle that divides the chest from the abdomen. Picture the lungs as two large inflated balloons within a barrel, their mouths connected to the outside through a Y tube. If all of the air outside of the balloons but inside of the barrel is removed, the balloons will inflate. If the barrel enlarges, so must the balloons. This is exactly what happens inside the chest, where the lungs reside, connected to the outside by a tube called the trachea. The outside surface of the lungs and the inside surface of the chest are covered with a smooth, moist mucosal membrane, much as are the tongue and cheeks within the mouth. This membrane is called the pleura, and the space between the lungs and the chest wall is called the pleural space. If a hole is made in the barrel, then the balloons inside it will collapse; if a hole is made in the chest wall, then collapse of the lung on that side ensues as air enters the pleural space. Air may also enter the pleural space from a leak in the lung, and in this case collapse also occurs. Regardless of the source of the air, air in the pleural space is termed pneumothorax, and pulmonary collapse is an inevitable result of pneumothorax.

In 1696, Giorgio Baglivi, a physician in Rome, reported to his colleagues that a patient of his with tuberculosis had dramatically improved following a sword wound to his chest that resulted in a pneumothorax. Three years later, a similar happening was described by the French physician de Blegny.[3] Dr. James Carson, a Scottish physician practicing in Liverpool, England in the early decades of the nineteenth century, was the first person to give serious thought to inducing pneumothoraces as a therapeutic modality. He conducted experiments on rabbits, demonstrating that a pneumothorax on one side was tolerated but that when a pneumothorax was induced on both sides it was invariably fatal. It was as though the balloon-lungs were enclosed within a securely partitioned barrel-thorax. Loss of pressure on one side meant lung collapse only on that side.

Carson convinced two of his patients to permit a surgeon to make wounds in their chests for the purpose of creating a pneumothorax. The procedure failed, although the patients were unharmed, because the lungs did not collapse. It now seems clear that Carson's patients had sufficient pleural disease so that the pleural space was extensively scarred. Collapse did not occur because the lungs were held in expansion by pleural scarring; the balloons were glued to the barrel. In 1834, F.H. Ramadge, an Irish contemporary of Carson practicing in London and probably aware of Carson's efforts, induced a pneumothorax in a tuberculous patient and reported that the patient was cured.[4]

Carlo Forlanini was the father of induced pneumothoraces for the treatment of tuberculosis. In 1882 he reported his review of prior experience with attempts to use pneumothorax therapeutically, and he concluded it was not a sufficiently safe procedure to be accepted. However, his interest was high, and he undertook a series of animal experiments that ultimately convinced him that lung collapse was feasible and that it could safely be done not simply by creating an opening in the chest wall but by introducing air with a syringe into the pleural space. On October 16, 1894 he induced a pneumothorax by injecting filtered air into the pleural space of a seventeen year old girl whom he described as having "fever, amenorrhea, and abundant expectoration, containing numerous tubercle bacilli. The disease was in a far advanced stage in the right lung with classical signs of cavity in the infraclavicular and scapular regions. The left lung was normal . . ." The pneumothorax was well tolerated by Forlanini's patient, and after four months he noted that she was much improved and that "cough and expectoration lessened, and she had gained weight and had fewer tubercle bacilli in her sputum."[5] Forlanini's procedure for introducing air into the pleural space was rapidly accepted in Europe and came into use in North America about fifteen years later.

John B. Murphy was a surgeon practicing in Chicago at the end of the nineteenth century. A feisty, bombastic, and self-centered individual who was disliked by many of his medical contemporaries, he was called the "Stormy Petrel of Surgery" by some of his peers.[6] At Chicago's Haymarket Riot in 1886, he found himself ministering to policemen wounded by a bomb thrown into their midst. He revelled in the extensive newspaper publicity given to his actions on behalf of the wounded. Later, he similarly encouraged newspaper reporters as they headlined news reports of his papers presented to medical meetings, "Cure of Consumption." Murphy became aware of Forlanini's work in Italy, and he sent his assistant, William Lemke, to Rome to learn the technique, and soon the two surgeons were reporting increasing numbers of patients successfully treated. In 1898, Murphy devised an apparatus consisting of bottles connected by tubes that allowed for the injections of measured amounts of air under controlled pressure. Murphy's device was the forerunner of later pneumothorax machines that were widely used as the procedure gained popularity.

The discovery of Xrays and the introduction of chest radiology early in the twentieth century, made it possible to identify patients with unilateral tuberculosis, especially unilateral tuberculous cavities, and apparently normal pleura. These patients were amenable to pneumothorax and were thought most likely to benefit from the procedure. Doctors felt more comfortable in recommending this treatment to their patients. The controversial Murphy probably also deserves credit for first emphasizing the importance of radiographic examinations in selecting patients for the use of pneumothorax therapy.

John Alexander, considered by many to be the father of thoracic surgery in America and author of the first American text on this subject, was a victim of tuberculosis. Suffering from Pott's disease, the destructive form of tuberculosis leading to deformity of the spine that is so readily identified in ancient mummies, he found himself at Saranac Lake in 1922, encased in a body cast intended to put his spine at rest and minimize deformity while allowing healing.[7] In his text, which he wrote during his confinement, he embraced the use of pneumothorax, thus bringing it into the mainstream of thoracic surgery.

Over the next quarter century, induced pneumothorax was used to treat some one hundred thousand patients with pulmonary tuberculosis, Edward Livingston Trudeau among them. Benefit was described in many, but no rigorous study of the results of the now widely accepted procedure was ever conducted. Moreover, it became increasingly apparent that there were some hazards associated with inducing pneumothoraces. The risks included inadvertent injection of air into a blood vessel, which could be fatal, infection of the pleural space either with tubercle bacilli or other germs, and bleeding. In some patients, attempts to induce a pneumothorax were unsuccessful because of pleural inflammation and scarring that prevented collapse of the lung. As Franz Kafka approached death from his tuberculosis in 1924, he wrote with remorse that his doctors considered him to be too ill to tolerate the procedure.[8]

So convinced of the benefit of lung collapse were the medical practitioners of the day that they set about looking for alternatives to pneumothorax that might be safer and that might be applied to more patients. Air was injected into the abdomen of some patients in a procedure termed pneumoperitoneum. This air was intended to force the diaphragm upward, thus compressing the lower lung lobes. For other patients, the diaphragm was brought into its resting elevated position by crushing a phrenic nerve. All muscles are controlled by nerves, and the phrenic nerves control the diaphragm. These two large nerves, right and left, leave the spinal cord high in neck and then make their way through the chest to the diaphragm on each side. A minor surgical procedure in the neck can expose these nerves, and the diaphragm can be paralyzed by crushing the nerve at this point.

Eric Blair, better known by his nom de plume, George Orwell, was ill with tuberculosis during much of his adult life. In 1938 he finally agreed to enter the hospital after a major episode of hemoptysis. He had a large tuberculous cavity in his left lung. A phrenic crush failed to arrest the disease, and he received a pneumoperitoneum. His tuberculosis did not improve, however. Later, he was started on newly discovered drugs for treatment, but he did not tolerate them. Orwell is probably best remembered for his great satirical novel *Nineteen Eighty-Four*. He struggled with advanced disease as he completed this work, and he died of tuberculosis in 1950 at the age of forty-six.[9]

Removal of ribs had long been known to surgeons as a technique for the treatment of some forms of pleural infections. Based on this prior experience, the idea of removing portions of ribs to reshape the chest wall and collapse underlying tuberculous lung was not a radical idea.

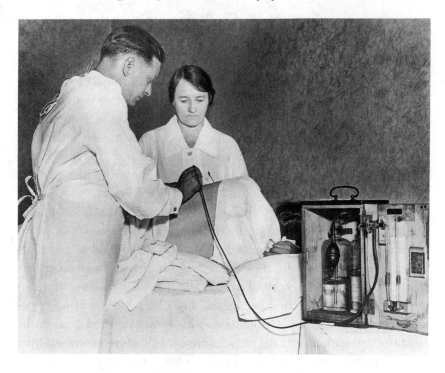

Figure 22.1. Injection of air into the pleural space of a patient with a pneumothorax induced to produce collapse of a lung affected by tuberculosis. A pneumothorax machine of the type invented by John Murphy is seen at lower right. Photograph courtesy of the American Lung Association.

The surgical procedure designed to accomplish the reshaping of the chest is termed thoracoplasty. It was probably first done by the Swiss surgeon De Cérenville in 1885. Ludloff Brauer, a Norwegian internist, and P. L. Friedrich, his surgical colleague, began using the technique and during the next decade introduced a number of important modifications.[10] The procedure they developed involved removing ribs in stages, two or three at a time, while leaving the fibrous covering of the ribs in place. After this procedure, ribs regenerated in their new position, creating a stable, reconfigured chest wall with diseased lung permanently collapsed beneath it. Because the collar bone supporting the shoulder was left in place, the disfigurement of the patient was not excessive and not readily apparent when the patient was fully clothed.

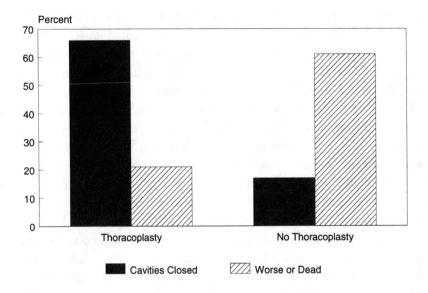

Figure 22.2. Outcome of patients for whom thoracoplasty was recommended for closure of tuberculous cavities and who either accepted and underwent the procedure or refused and did not have thoracoplasties. It is apparent that the prognosis of cavitary tuberculosis in patients who were deemed suitable candidates for thoracoplasty was greatly improved by this operation. Data from Meade RH. A history of thoracic surgery. Springfield, IL: Charles C. Thomas Publisher, 1961:126-127.

But permanent deformity resulted. Patients accepted it in hopes of cure of their dread disease.

Thoracoplasty was slow to win acceptance among American surgeons. However, during the 1930s it gained increasing acceptance. In 1937, Cleveland physicians Sidney Wolpaw, an internist with an interest in tuberculosis, and Samuel Freedlander, a thoracic surgeon, described the outcome of one hundred and fifty-three patients for whom thoracoplasty was recommended between 1932 and 1934. Eighty-five of the patients accepted the procedure, and their results were compared with those of the fifty-eight who refused. In 1936, two to four years later, sixty-six percent of those treated had closed their tuberculous cavities; only seventeen percent of those who refused had closed their cavities. Twenty-one percent of those operated upon were worse or dead; sixty-one percent of those not receiving thoracoplasty were worse or dead.[11] The benefit of thoracoplasty was dramatically apparent. Figure 22.2 presents these results graphically. Similar results were reported by other surgeons in the subsequent years, and this procedure became an accepted manner of dealing with cavitary tuberculosis. Indeed, patients with unilateral cavities considered themselves fortunate because they were suitable candidates for this mutilating surgery.

Thoracoplasty was not an unmixed blessing. The procedure itself was hazardous. To avoid shock, ribs had to be resected piecemeal, meaning several operations. Bleeding was a problem. And patients sometimes spread their disease to the lung on the other side during the operation. Surgeons of the 1930s devised methods for separating the pleura from the chest wall and introducing material into the space thus created. In this way, the underlying lung could be collapsed without actually removing ribs or deforming the chest wall. Paraffin was initially inserted into this space; later grafts of muscle and fat were used. In 1948, plastic balls about the size of ping pong balls came into use for this purpose. These procedures, called plombage or extrapleural plombage, were safer than thoracoplasty, but they were complicated by problems many years later of erosion of the plombage material through the pleural membrane and into the underlying collapsed lung.

Like bed rest, collapse therapies have now been consigned to history, displaced by the more effective drug treatment that we will consider in the next chapters. Although never subjected to the type of rigorous evaluation that we now demand of new therapies, they clearly aided certain patients. They also had their costs, including risks associated with the surgical procedures, loss of lung function, increased burden on the heart, and disfigurement. In the great war against tuberculosis, they represented battles won by some patients, but hardly moments of great victory.

23

Magic Bullet

The scientific knowledge gained during the past decade, it is said, equals or exceeds that of the previous century; that gained during the past century that of the previous millennium; that of the past millennium that of all history. One must stand in awe of this hurtling race to new knowledge. One must ask what further knowledge frontiers will remain tomorrow. Nowhere has this accelerating scientific explosion been more dramatic than in the discovery of new disease treatments.

Koch's discovery that tuberculosis is caused by a specific germ (Chapter 9) led almost immediately to attempts to find agents that would attack the infecting bacillus. Koch, as we have learned, focused his thoughts on ways to stimulate the body's immune defense mechanisms to destroy tubercle bacilli. His tuberculin failed, as have other attempts at stimulation of immunity in the face of established disease. But the seed of another idea was germinating within the new science of microbiology. If a dye could selectively stain tubercle bacilli and not the surrounding human tissues, as Koch and later Ehrlich had observed, then might there not be an agent that would attack tubercle bacilli, kill or weaken them, but not attack humans? Could not the specificity seen in dye staining equally be present in drug actions? Quinine appeared to offer something of this sort in curing malaria. Moreover, compounds of certain metals—arsenic, mercury, bismuth—appeared to attack the germ causing syphilis without seriously harming the person ill with this disease. Karen Blixen left her farm in Africa at the foot of the Ngong Hills to return to Europe to receive these metal injections. Both quinine and metals were tried for tuberculosis, but with little benefit. Then, in the 1932, came prontosil, a red dye that killed many bacteria, the discovery of Gerhardt Domagk and his colleagues at Bayer, the German dye and chemical giant. Three years later scientists at the Pasteur Institute in

Paris found the active moiety of prontosil to be sulfonilamide, and the sulfonamides were born. Sulfonamides proved to be effective against many of the bacteria causing human infections, and they ushered in the modern era of chemotherapy for infections. In the early 1940s the miraculous penicillin joined the fray.[1]

These new wonder drugs did not attack tubercle bacilli. However, that short-coming did not dampen the ardor of the medical community seeking a magic bullet capable of selectively destroying the pernicious and pervasive microbe that caused tuberculosis. Rather, it stimulated further search. The great hero of this search was Selman A. Waksman.

Selman Abraham Waksman was born on July 22, 1888 in a mud and thatch hovel in the Ukrainian steppes village of Novaia-Priluka.[2] His mother, Fradia, a devout Jewess, dedicated her son to God and named him for the great King Solomon. She nurtured him through his boyhood, encouraged his scholarly bent, and lavished affection upon him. His father, Jacob, struggling to provide sustenance for his family, was often absent. Although remembered by Waksman as kind and loving, he was not the important, character-shaping parent that both his mother and his maternal grandmother were. Waksman's only sibling, a younger sister, died at the age of two of diphtheria.

The family was devoutly Jewish, and Waksman's boyhood was dominated by his religion and by his growing love for the agrarian land in which he lived. He proved to be a gifted student, but in the Ukraine of his time, his Jewish background handicapped him as he sought acceptance to a gymnasium. Ultimately, he pursued his education as an irregular student in Odesa and Vinnytsya.

With his secondary education completed, Waksman returned to his village in 1909 and began supporting himself as a tutor. That summer his mother died of an acute intestinal obstruction, for which medical care was not available locally. The young man was devastated. The following spring he failed to gain entrance to one of the few positions open to Jews at the university in Odesa. Life in his homeland seemed to offer no opportunities for him, particularly since he was bent on pursuing a career of scholarship. He decided to emigrate to America, where he had cousins, to, in his words, "begin life anew and forget the old world."[3]

Waksman arrived in Philadelphia on November 2, 1910. He was met by two of his cousins. One of them Mendel Kornblatt, owned a farm in Metuchen, New Jersey, and Waksman was soon installed as a worker on the Kornblatt farm. But further education was the young man's goal, and before long he set out to explore his opportunities. He was admitted to the College of Physicians and Surgeons of Columbia University in New York, Edward Livingston Trudeau's alma mater, but felt he could not afford the high cost of tuition. He visited Rutgers College in nearby New Brunswick, and there he met Professor Jacob G. Lipman. Lipman, also a Russian immigrant and then head of the Department of Bacteriology, was to have a profound influence on Waksman. Lipman encouraged him and urged him to pursue his emerging interests in soil microbiology. Importantly, Rutgers offered him a scholarship.

For the next two and one-half years, Waksman lived and worked on the Kornblatt farm, learning the fundamentals of agriculture in a practical sense while his academic studies introduced him to the science underlying plant and soil phenomena. At the end of his sophomore year, Waksman moved to an old farmhouse on the Rutgers College Farm grounds. He received a modest stipend for assisting in studies of plant nutrition and plant genetics. He earned additional money as a night watchman and as an assistant in the Poultry Department, a position that included the added benefit of the opportunity to purchase cracked eggs at eleven cents a dozen. His studies progressed, and under the tutelage of Dr. Lipman he began to study a particular group of fungal soil microbes known as actinomycetes. Waksman's life was happy, the more so because his sweetheart from his homeland, Bobili, emigrated to New York. Waksman traveled to that city on weekends to continue his courtship of her.

Waksman was elected to Phi Beta Kappa and graduated from Rutgers in 1915 and began studies for a masters degree in microbiology under Dr. Lipman. He wrote his first scientific paper, "Bacteria, Actinomyces, and Fungi of the Soil." It was read by Dr. Lipman before the annual meeting of the Society of American Bacteriologists in December 1915, but it was not published. An abstract was printed in the Journal of Bacteriology. Other papers followed and were published.

In the summer of 1916, Waksman received his masters degree, married Bobili, and moved to the University of California at Berkeley to enter a Ph.D. program with Dr. T.B. Robertson, a biochemist. Waksman felt that increasing his knowledge of biochemistry would be important to a career in soil microbiology, his now firmly-fixed goal. While life was pleasant in California, it was less productive scientifically and more difficult financially than the young scientist had hoped it would be. He found it necessary to take a job at Cutter laboratories supervising the preparation of bacteriological media. When the opportunity presented itself to return to Rutgers as a Lecturer in Dr. Lipman's Department of Soil Microbiology in 1918, Waksman readily accepted.

The next two decades were happy and extraordinarily productive ones for Selman Waksman. His research went well and he became a recognized expert on the microorganisms that inhabit soil and on their role in soil ecology. He rose through the academic ranks to become a Professor and head of his own research group and laboratory. He made several trips to Europe to participate in scientific congresses and consult with other leaders in the emerging science of microbiology, and he became a leader in international scientific societies. The National Academy of Sciences honored him by election to its august membership. His marriage was happy, and his only son, Byron, was emerging as a talented young man headed for a career in science.[4] A return visit to Priluka, his Ukrainian birthplace, in 1924 was disheartening, however, for the social turmoil of the Russian revolution had left that village a site of destitution and poverty.

Waksman consulted with industry on the problems of composting and the commercial uses of peat. One early consultancy, which not only aided his personal finances as he struggled to establish himself and his family again in New Jersey but also broadened his thinking, was with Takamine Laboratories. This company, whose founder was a distinguished Japanese emigrant chemist also remembered for making the initial gift of three hundred of the cherry trees that now adorn the Potomac River basin in Washington, was engaged in manufacturing Salvarsan, a compound of arsenic used for the treatment of syphilis. For the first time, Waksman was asked to think about the effect that drugs could have on infection, a new challenge for him.

World War II enveloped the world. Waksman was initially called upon to study methods of reducing the fouling of ships bottoms. The attack on Pearl Harbor made it apparent that American troops would become engaged in the South Pacific, and Waksman's knowledge of soil fungi was sought for help in dealing with both the health problems of American troops and the maintenance problems of American equipment presented by fungus-rich tropical environments. Soon, Waksman, now President of the American Society of Bacteriologists, was appointed Chairman of the War Committee on Bacteriology.

The war effort provided stimulus for a new line of research, for the exploration of new ideas and a new field of investigation that had begun to intrigue Waksman, for the study of antibiotics. Antibiotics. Wonder drugs. In all the history of medicine, two great advances stand out as having had more impact on disease than any other. The first was immunization, ushered in by Jenner and Pasteur (Chapter 15); the second antibiotics. Antibiotics are substances produced by one microorganism that kill or impair the growth of other microorganisms. Some, although not all, are so specific in their action that they do not harm humans and thus can be used in the treatment of infections.

Waksman coined the term antibiotic, and he soon became a leader in this field of science. Penicillin, Fleming's, Florey's, and Chain's discovery in Britain and the first antibiotic to come into widespread medical use, was limited in its spectrum of activity. René Dubos, who earned his Ph.D. with Waksman and developed the fundamental methods for identifying antibiotics produced by soil microbes in Waksman's laboratory before moving to the Rockefeller Institute, had discovered gramicidin. Too toxic to be ingested, this early antibiotic was widely used for external applications.

Waksman's attention was increasingly drawn to soil actinomycetes, the organisms so familiar to him. Several antibiotics with exciting microbe-killing capabilities were found by Waksman's laboratory team, but they all were too toxic for human use. The search continued and the work proliferated. Financial support was provided by foundations and drug companies, notably including Merck and Company, that negotiated agreements with Rutgers University. Scientists and students flocked to Waksman's laboratory, and soon he had a large team working under his direction. Waksman's son Byron, then a medical student, urged him to seek agents active against the tubercle bacillus.[5]

In August 1943, a poultry pathologist at an agricultural station in New Jersey isolated an actinomycete from the throat of a sick chicken

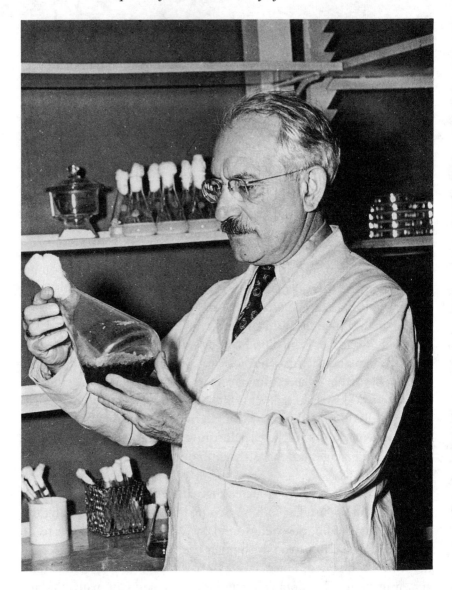

Figure 23.1. Selman Waksman in his laboratory in November 1947, four years after the discovery of streptomycin. Photograph courtesy of the American Lung Association.

brought to the station by a New Jersey poultry farmer. The culture of this organism was forwarded to Waksman, and thence to one of his graduate students, Albert Schatz. Schatz had joined the laboratory only two months earlier and had been set by Waksman on the task of searching for new antibiotics. Schatz was a prodigious worker. Soon, he and a coworker, Elizabeth Bugie, had identified the organism as *Streptomyces griseus*, a soil actinomycete originally described by Waksman in 1919 and only recently reclassified and given its current name. From this strain and from a similar strain isolated from a heavily manured field, they isolated a new antibiotic, which they named streptomycin. Within an incredibly short four months, they had compared it with other known antibiotics and tested it for its activity against twenty-two different bacteria.[6] It displayed remarkable antibiotic activity against several microorganisms, including a number not touched by penicillin or sulfonamides. Among these was the tubercle bacillus. Furthermore, it was less toxic in animals than the antibiotics previously isolated from actinomycetes by Waksman's laboratory group.

The work in Waksman's laboratory attracted the attention of Drs. H. Corwin Hinshaw and William H. Feldman at the Mayo Clinic. These two scientists knew little of antibiotics, but they were ardent students of tuberculosis. Hinshaw was a distinguished academic pulmonary physician, devoted to learning about tuberculosis from the study of his patients. Feldman was an experimentalist, trained as a veterinary microbiologist, and equally devoted to learning more about this important disease. Intrigued by Waksman's early reports of antibiotics from actinomycetes, Feldman visited Waksman's laboratory at Rutgers in November 1943, during the time when Albert Schatz was diligently conducting experiments with the newly discovered streptomycin. Later, Waksman traveled to the Mayo Clinic in Rochester, Minnesota in October 1944 to present a seminar at that prestigious institution.[7] Waksman then sent a supply of crude streptomycin containing less than six percent of the active drug to the two Minnesotans. Using this material, they conducted the first studies of the drug in animals. Soon, their supplies were augmented by further amounts of more highly purified drug from Merck and Company, for this drug manufacturer, which had collaborated with Waksman for several years, was now engaged in the production of streptomycin.

Working without assistance and getting up at night to inject their guinea pigs every three hours for six weeks, Feldman and Hinshaw conducted carefully controlled experiments. The results were dramatic. In the first experiment, completed in June 1944, tuberculous infection progressed in all of four infected guinea pigs that were not treated, and two of them died. All four guinea pigs given streptomycin lived and their infections disappeared. Further larger experiments were equally dramatic. There was no doubt in the two medical scientists' minds. Streptomycin cured tuberculous guinea pigs.[8]

A twenty-one year-old woman, whom history records only as Patricia T., was admitted to the Mineral Springs Sanatorium in Cannon Falls, Minnesota in July 1943 with far advanced tuberculosis. A year of sanatorium care produced some improvement, but in October 1944, she worsened. Her fever, night sweats, and cough returned. Her weight dropped to seventy-five pounds. Her chest radiograph showed progression of her disease and increased cavitation in the right upper lobe. The first stage of a planned multi-stage thoracoplasty was performed on November 1, 1944. It was followed by the dreaded complication of spread to the other lung. Dr. Karl F. Pfuetze, her doctor, consulted with Dr. Hinshaw. The two physicians were sure the young woman would die if the present course continued, and they proposed to her that she become the first person to be treated with streptomycin. The frightened young woman was eager to accept the challenge; she probably thought little about the historic import of her decision.[9]

Streptomycin injections were given to Patricia T. beginning on November 20, 1944. The drug was appropriated from that supplied for the guinea pig studies. Injections were given every three hours. They were painful, and they induced unpleasant reactions including pain, fever, and headache. The dose of active drug given amounted to about one-tenth to one-fifth of what was later found to be the optimal amount for treatment. After ten days, the injections were stopped to allow the patient to recover from the painful reactions. They were restarted for another ten days a month later. A chest radiograph discouragingly showed no change. Then, more highly purified drug became available, and on January 13, 1945 treatment was reinstituted, with daily doses approximating those that later came to be standard for therapy and continued for forty-five days. Patricia T. began to improve. The number of tubercle bacilli in her sputum decreased. The fresh disease in her left lung, which had developed after her attempted thoracoplasty, cleared up completely. Patricia T. was on the way to recovery, and the modern tuberculosis chemotherapy era had begun. Streptomycin was a magic bullet.

Patricia T. remained in the sanatorium at Cannon Falls for two more years. Three additional operations completed the planned thoracoplasty to close the cavities in her right lung. She went home on July 13, 1947, her diseased now arrested. She married and had three healthy children in 1950, 1952, and 1954. A follow-up examination in August 1954 demonstrated that her tuberculosis remained inactive.

Other patients soon followed; in September 1945, Drs. Hinshaw and Feldman reported the results of treatment of thirty-four patients.[10] A year later the number of patients they had treated had grown to one hundred.[11] They were cautiously optimistic about the promise of the new drug. Waksman and Merck and Company provided additional supplies to many investigators, and the favorable results in Minnesota were duplicated throughout the country. Acceptance of this treatment came rapidly. By 1953, ten thousand scientific papers and twenty books devoted to streptomycin had been published. More than a score of companies were producing the drug.

Streptomycin was slow to reach Europe, and in Great Britain, supplies of streptomycin were extremely limited. In September 1946, a special committee of the British Medical Research Council met to plan the best use to be made of the small available supply of the new wonder drug. From their efforts emerged a clinical trial that remains to this day the undisputed standard of excellence in such clinical investigations.[12] It is the model for today's trials of chemotherapeutic agents for treating cancer. Carefully selected patients were randomly assigned to receive or not receive the new antibiotic for four months, and the experts who subsequently evaluated the results were blinded to the therapy. What was the outcome of this study? The results are depicted in Figure 23.2. After six months, clinical improvement was noted in forty of the fifty-five patients who received streptomycin and in twenty-six of the fifty-two who did not. The chest radiographs improved in thirty-eight of the treated persons and in seventeen of the untreated control patients. Four of the fifty-five streptomycin-treated patients died; fourteen of the fifty-two control subjects died. The microbiologic results were less dramatic.

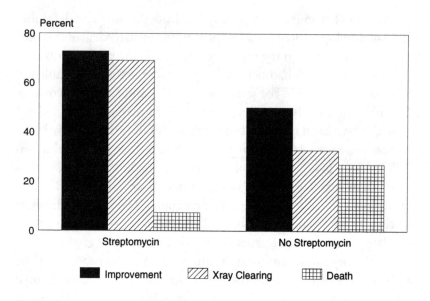

Figure 23.2. Results of the British Medical Research Council streptomycin trial. With respect to percent of patients who were assessed as having clinical improvement, radiographic (Xray) clearing, and survival at six months after initiation of therapy, there was a clear difference between the streptomycin group and the control subjects who were hospitalized under similar conditions but not given streptomycin. Data from Medical Research Council. Streptomycin treatment of pulmonary tuberculosis. Brit Med J 1948; 2:769-82.

At the end of six months, only eight treated patients had completely cleared tubercle bacilli from their sputum. Two control patients had also achieved this desired result. When a final evaluation was completed one year after the start of treatment, thirty-one of the fifty-five patients given streptomycin were improved; twelve had died. Only sixteen of the fifty-two control subjects were improved, and twenty-four had died. Streptomycin was unequivocally of benefit, but it would not be a miracle-producing drug for all sufferers from tuberculosis.

Fame followed quickly for Waksman. Honor followed honor. He received the prestigious Lasker Award, and in 1952 Selman Abraham Waksman was awarded the Nobel Prize in Physiology and Medicine. In his acceptance speech, Waksman noted, "From the moment he is born to the moment he dies, man is subject to the activities of microbes. Some are injurious and others are beneficial. The latter have made recently a great contribution to mankind by producing the antibiotics. There has thus been placed in the hands of the medical profession one of the greatest tools for combating infectious diseases of man and of animals."[13]

What could mar the triumph of Selman Waksman? The cloud on his horizon was none other than Albert Schatz, the diligent graduate student who actually performed most of the laboratory experiments leading to the isolation of streptomycin. When the two and one-half percent royalties on streptomycin sales began to enrich Rutgers University and Waksman, who originally received one-fifth of the royalties, later one-tenth, Schatz, who received nothing, filed a law suit.[14] He was first author on the original publication, and his name was on the patent application as one of the inventors. He felt he deserved a share of the income and that he had been coerced into assigning all of his interests to Rutgers University. Rutgers settled the suit before it went to trial for one-quarter of a million dollars. Additional payments were made to other members of Waksman's laboratory team. In later years, the still embittered Schatz would protest, sometimes stridently, that he too should have been recognized by the Nobel Prize Committee.

I do not intend to join in the argument in which many authors have chosen to take sides. Schatz was a student. He had arrived in the laboratory only two months before he was given the remarkable culture from the throat of a sick chicken. He did most of the actual work. That is undisputed. Waksman was the expert. No one can dispute that. Waksman had the vision, knowledge, and ideas and had had them building in his brain for more than a decade. He had coined the very word antibiotic, and he was the outstanding microbiologist of his era. He and other members of his group, including René Dubos, had developed the methods of investigation that Schatz used so assiduously and effectively. Schatz felt that he suffered abasement in the laboratory. So also had Waksman in his graduate student days, and Schatz's life was little different from that of other graduate students in that day. Waksman had revered Jacob Lipman, his professor and mentor, and at his insistence the new institute being built at Rutgers with the royalties from streptomycin was to be named not for Waksman but for Lipman.

Perhaps Schatz was in lesser awe of Waksman. Both men in their separate ways contributed to the conquest of tuberculosis. So also did Hinshaw and Feldman at the Mayo Clinic. So also did Dubos. So also— and least honored today of all—did the courageous Patricia T.

24

Microbe Killers

Eric Martin Blair, who later adopted the name George Orwell, was born in 1903 in India, the son of a British civil servant. He is remembered today as a champion of liberal causes, an outspoken opponent of fascism, political leftist, and the author of great satirical novels, including *Animal Farm* and *Nineteen Eighty-Four.* He had tuberculosis and was treated with streptomycin. However, the new wonder drug did not save his life.[1]

As an infant, Orwell was sickly with bronchitis. As an adult he was given the diagnosis of pneumonia on several occasions, and in 1938, after returning from fighting in the Spanish Civil War, he was first told he had tuberculosis. His disease progressed in the stuttering, remitting and relapsing fashion typical of tuberculosis. He continued to write, but he was never again free of illness and his work and life were interrupted by repeated hospitalizations. *Nineteen Eighty-Four* was completed as he approached his death.

In 1948 he underwent a phrenic crush to paralyze his left diaphragm and a pneumoperitoneum. These procedures were undertaken in an attempt to promote healing of the cavitary disease in his left lung (Chapter 22). Streptomycin had become available in the United States, but there was none in Britain. Orwell contacted his American friend, David Astor, who obtained the drug for him. Within two months, he was feeling better, but a severe dermatitis was caused by the streptomycin. Reading his accounts of this skin problem, it is clear that he had an exfoliative dermatitis and probably the potentially fatal Stevens-Johnson syndrome, a drug reaction not frequently associated with streptomycin. Wisely, his doctors discontinued the streptomycin treatment.[2]

Hoping for relief in the magic mountains, Orwell went to Switzerland in January 1950. There he fell victim to the Captain of Death on

January 21, 1950, at the age of forty-six. Streptomycin failed him, not because it did not attack his tubercle bacilli but because his body was unable to tolerate the new drug.

Among the limitations of streptomycin—including its toxicity for Orwell and other patients, the fact that it failed to cure some with chronic and advanced disease, and a relapse rate of approximately ten percent after successful treatment—none was more troubling than the development of a new breed of tuberculosis germs with resistance to the wonder drug antibiotic. Where did this drug resistance come from? In fact, tuberculosis germs and other microbes, like all living beings, are subject to the laws of natural selection and evolution observed by Charles Darwin among finches in the Galapagos Islands. Indeed, modern scientists find bacteria, with their very short generation times, ideal organisms for the study of evolutionary mechanisms.

The average patient with active tuberculosis probably harbors several hundred million to one billion individual tuberculosis germs. Of these germs, perhaps one in ten thousand carries a genetic mutation making it resistant to any given tuberculosis-fighting drug. That is not very many of these troublesome mutants, or is it? A bit of division reveals that there are approximately one thousand to ten thousand drug-resistant tuberculosis germs in the average patient we are considering. Now let us add a second and different drug, equally effective, and with a similar likelihood that one in ten thousand bacilli are resistant to it. Now our patient is likely to harbor at most only one bacterium resistant to both drugs. The answer is obvious. Tuberculosis patients should be treated simultaneously with two or even three equally effective antituberculosis drugs. Selman Waksman's magic bullet of streptomycin needed to be supplemented by an arsenal of several other potent medicines.

The giant pharmaceutical companies of Germany developed sulfonamides during the 1930s and 1940s. Not derived from other microorganisms and hence not fitting Waksman's definition of antibiotic, they were none-the-less capable of killing many disease-producing bacteria. But these agents did not affect tubercle bacilli. It was hard for German pharmacologists to understand why they did not, and so a search was launched in many laboratories for similar or related drugs that would take on tuberculosis.[3] Two drugs came to the fore, a semithiocarbazone now known as thioacetazone, and para-aminosalicylic acid, widely known by its initials, PAS. Soon, these drugs were being given together with streptomycin, and resistance to the antibiotic became a less frequently encountered problem. However, both of these drugs were weaklings in killing power compared to streptomycin, in medical terms, bacteriostatic rather than bactericidal. Moreover, both drugs were toxic and difficult for patients to take. Something better was needed. The search continued.

Independently, unaware of one another's activities, and almost simultaneously, scientists at three large pharmaceutical companies, Bayer, in Germany, Squibb, and Hoffman-La Roche, both in the United States, pursued their search for a new microbe killer molecule and found the same prize. Testing one variation after another of molecules with structures related to that of PAS and thioacetazone, all three groups of workers hit upon isonicotinic hydrazide, soon to be renamed isoniazid or, more simply, INH. More than ten times more potent than any previously tested drug and apparently nontoxic, the promise of INH was extraordinary. Moreover, INH had been described in a published report by chemists many years earlier. INH could not be patented. Anyone could make it and sell it, and it was not difficult or expensive to produce.

Not surprisingly, there was a race to test this new apparent wonder drug in patients with tuberculosis. The front runners in this race were Irving J. Selikoff, Edward H. Robitzek, and George G. Ornstein, three physicians working at the Sea View Hospital, a tuberculosis sanatorium in New York. In the summer of 1951, Hoffman-La Roche gave them a supply of isoniazid and a very closely related compound, iproniazid. They made a few preliminary investigations of toxicity and dosing, and on October 2, 1951 they were ready to begin. They selected one hundred and seventy-five patients with extensive active tuberculosis. All had been previously treated with currently accepted methods and had failed to improve. Most were toxic with their disease. All faced dismal futures.

Isoniazid was given to sixty-five of these desperately ill patients, iproniazid to one hundred and one, and a combination of iproniazid and streptomycin to nine.[4] The results were dramatic, and unlike anything seen previously in the treatment of tuberculosis. Patients temperatures fell to normal over the course of one to three weeks. "We have seen instances," wrote Selikoff and his colleagues, "of reversal to normal temperature within twenty-four hours in patients who had been continuously febrile for several months."[5] Appetite returned, sometimes ravenously, with weight returning to normal or even above normal levels within two to three months in all patients. Similarly, cough, the most characteristic symptom of phthisis, disappeared, and tubercle bacilli disappeared from the sputum of most patients. Clearing of disease apparent on chest radiographs occurred within two to three months in two-thirds of the treated patients. Toxicity from the two hydrazide drugs was minimal, but greater with iproniazid than isoniazid. Results such as these were totally unprecedented in the history of tuberculosis. As word reached the public, there was jubilation and widespread hope that a miracle cure was finally at hand. *Life* magazine featured a picture of patients treated with INH dancing in the corridors of Sea View Hospital.

Extraordinarily effective, extremely well tolerated, and inexpensive, isoniazid rapidly became the linchpin of tuberculosis therapy. Because of the need to prevent the emergence of drug-resistant mutant tubercle bacilli, other drugs were used in combination with isoniazid. Streptomycin was highly effective in this role, but it had to be given by injection and had significant toxicity. PAS was commonly used, although it was difficult for patients to tolerate. A new drug, ethambutol, was expensive, but much easier to take, and it soon replaced PAS. Thioacetazone became the second drug most widely used in developing countries, favored because of its very low cost, despite some risk of toxicity. Eighteen to twenty-four months of two drug treatment cured most patients. The very term "arrested tuberculosis" disappeared from the medical lexicon.

The change in treatment of tuberculosis was rapid and dramatic. Within five years, rest therapy had been abandoned. In the late 1950s, the United States army conducted studies of patients who were entered into active exercise programs. I was an army physician working in an army chest hospital at that time, and all of my patients were enrolled in a study in which they were either allowed to set their own level of physical activity or sent to the base gymnasium to play basketball and do calisthenic exercises twice weekly. The exercise—a radical departure from previous treatment—improved the sense of well being and general health of these tuberculosis patients and did not interfere with the healing of their disease. To this day, however, I regret having participated in a decision to tell a long distance runner with tuberculosis not to compete in trials for the Olympic Games. Such strenuous exertion seemed too risky. Today, I would make a different decision.

In India, an additional potential benefit of isoniazid treatment of tuberculosis was imagined. Hospital beds were simply not available for most patients with tuberculosis. Was it necessary to hospitalize drug-treated patients at all, asked doctors in Madras? A study was designed, and one hundred and ninety-three newly diagnosed tuberculous patients with tubercle bacilli in their sputum were randomly assigned to treatment at home or treatment in a tuberculosis hospital for one year.[6] All patients were given isoniazid and PAS for one year. Hospitalized patients had the benefit of more rest and much more nutritious diets than those patients who stayed at home. Social workers visited the patients at home to be sure they took their medicines. Both groups of patients did extremely well, and there were no differences in the outcomes between the two groups. When reexamined five years after treatment had been started, eighty-two of the ninety-six patients treated at home and eighty-four of the ninety-seven hospitalized patients were alive, well, and free of tuberculosis.

What of the risk of contagion from patients kept at home? Would they infect others if left unhospitalized? The children and other household members of the Madras patients were also followed.[7] Among two hundred and fifty-six contacts of patients treated at home, twenty-four (nine percent) developed tuberculosis. Among two hundred and seventy-two contacts of hospitalized patients, thirty-eight (fourteen percent) developed tuberculosis. It was time to close tuberculosis hospitals!

Close them we did. Isoniazid became generally available to all tuberculosis patients in 1953. In that year, there were eight hundred and thirty-nine tuberculosis hospitals in the United States with more than one hundred and thirty thousand beds dedicated to consumptive patients.[8] One year later, in the fall of 1954 and scarcely more than three years after the first patient received isoniazid at Sea View Hospital, Trudeau's Adirondack Cottage Sanitarium in Saranac Lake announced it would close. By 1972, there were only four tuberculosis hospitals still open in America with four hundred and twenty beds. The rise in tuberculosis sanatoria and tuberculosis sanatorium beds in the United States during the first half of the twentieth century and the precipitous

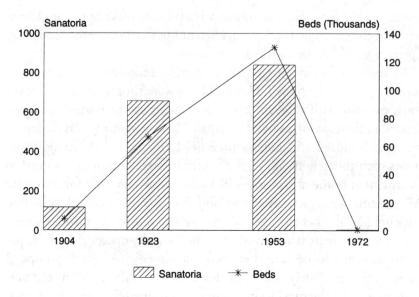

Figure 24.1. The rise and fall of tuberculosis sanatoria and sanatorium beds in the United States during the twentieth century. The rapid increase during the first half of the century was followed by an even more dramatic decline during the two decades following the introduction of isoniazid. Data from Davis AL. History of the sanatorium movement. In Rom WN, Garay SM, editors. Tuberculosis. Little, Brown and Company, New York, NY, 1996:35-54.

decline in these facilities following the introduction of isoniazid are depicted in Figure 24.1.

In the early 1970s a tuberculosis bed in New York City cost $97 per day; the cost of drugs for treating tuberculosis was $11.55 per day. The savings in direct hospital care costs in the United States for the fifteen year period 1954 to 1969 were nearly four billion dollars. During that same time period, the United States government allocated less than one-sixth of that amount to the National Institutes of Health for research and research training for all infectious diseases.[9] One would like to think that this experience would have convinced budget makers of the long term cost effectiveness of scientific research. However, history tells us otherwise.

Inevitably, tubercle bacilli resistant to isoniazid began to appear. It should have been no surprise to anyone. More microbe killers were needed, and scientific discovery responded to the need. In 1957 a new class of antibiotics known as rifamycins were isolated from *Streptomyces mediterranei* at the laboratories of Lepetit, a pharmaceutical company in Milan, Italy. Although promising, these agents needed to be administered by injection and they were so rapidly removed from the body by the liver that it was very difficult to achieve adequate drug levels for treatment. The Lepetit chemists modified the molecules of these new antibiotics, and from their efforts a new drug, rifampin, was born. Rifampin received its first clinical trials in Europe in the mid 1960s. In Belgium it was given to a small number of patients with chronic tuberculosis who had failed previous treatment and were considered "nearly hopeless." Dramatic improvement occurred in all the patients who received rifampin, and the drug was well tolerated. The first American trials of this new drug were presented to an excited audience at a scientific meeting sponsored by the Veterans Administration in January 1969.[10]

Modern knowledge of how best to use the new antibiotics came slowly. As we have already noted, bacteria resistant to one agent can be discouraged by using more than one drug at once. A series of elegant studies conducted in Asia, India, and Africa under the leadership of Wallace Fox and Dennis Mitchison of the British Medical Research Council established the general principles that guide all modern treatment.[11] Initially, multiple drugs are given, typically three, sometimes four. One or two months of this therapy results in rapid killing of most of the infecting tubercle bacilli. Several months of consolidation treatment, usually using isoniazid and one other drug, follows to kill all remaining tubercle bacilli and secure the cure.

While victory appears to be at hand, clouds remain on the horizon. First, there is the ever troublesome problem of the ability of the tubercle bacillus to mutate and allow drug-resistant strains to emerge. Next, even with the usual course of treatment now measured in months, it is difficult to insure that patients complete all of their prescribed therapy; failure to do so leads to relapse. Vivien Leigh, one of the most talented and beautiful actresses ever to grace the stage and movie screen, developed tuberculosis in 1945 at the age of thirty-one.[12] During six weeks of hospitalization her cough improved and she gained weight. Her doctor recommended that she go to a sanatorium for further treatment, but she refused. Through the rest of her life, the talented actress, who knew so many triumphs on the stage, was stalked by tuberculosis. Plagued also by manic-depressive disease and, perhaps as a manifestation of her mental illness, alcoholism, she continued to refuse treatment. New treatments became available, including streptomycin and isoniazid, but Vivien Leigh refused them. She died on July 7, 1967, a victim not only of tuberculosis but of her unwillingness or inability to accept treatment with the microbe killers that might have cured her.

Finally, we must not forget that the curative weapons we have to combat tuberculosis are not universally available. The cost of treatment programs and the drugs they depend on remains a barrier to bringing health and disease control to people in many of the impoverished countries of the world. It is in precisely those countries where the largest number of persons with tuberculosis cry out for help.

25

One One-Hundredth of an Ounce of Prevention

With effective curative drug treatment available for patients with tuberculosis and a vaccine, albeit of uncertain efficacy in hand for immunization, what further challenges remained for health scientists intent on conquering this dread disease? Once again, let us think back to the story of Eleanor Roosevelt (Chapter 5). Infected as a young woman, she developed her fatal disease late in life. Too late for vaccination, for she had already been infected. Beyond the reach of treatment, for her diagnosis was not made promptly and her disseminated disease progressed rapidly. What could have been done for her?

During the years when Eleanor Roosevelt was pursuing her extraordinary international career, Edith Lincoln was a pediatrician working in the Pediatric Chest Clinic at Bellevue Hospital in New York. Most of her patients had tuberculosis, and many of these children died of the disease to which their young age rendered them so susceptible. In 1954, she published a study of tuberculosis as it had been seen at that hospital prior to effective drug treatment and in the newly dawning drug treatment era.[1] From 1930 to 1946, the years preceding streptomycin, nine hundred and eighty tuberculous children were seen in her clinic, and twenty-one and one-half percent of them died of the disease. In the short interval of 1952 and 1953 after the introduction of isoniazid, one hundred and twenty-nine patients were seen, and only one and one-half percent of them died of tuberculosis. This great killer of children had been conquered.

In discussing her exciting results, Lincoln noted that many of the children who had died or who had been treated and saved from death had initially been seen with primary tuberculosis. That is, they had been brought to the clinic at an early time when infection had occurred but had not progressed to the chronic disease we know as tuberculosis. Drug therapy for those fortunate to have lived during the time when such treatment was available protected them from later development of lethal disease. Lincoln wrote, "If these observations are substantiated, it may radically change the present indications for specific therapy in primary tuberculosis. The use of isoniazid will have to be considered for every child with active primary tuberculosis and probably also for children with known recent conversion of tuberculin tests even if chest roentgenograms are normal."[2]

Lincoln's idea was a radical one. She suggested that all persons—all children, at least—with positive tuberculin skin tests might benefit from isoniazid treatment even before they became clinically ill and even though many of them would never develop disease. Lincoln did more than publish her idea in a medical journal; she took it to her colleagues at the United States Public Health Service. As the idea was scrutinized by tuberculosis physicians and public health officials, it became more and more attractive. Isoniazid was cheap and exceptionally nontoxic. Because infected but nondiseased individuals generally harbored no more than about one hundred tubercle bacilli, the one in ten thousand drug-resistant microbes were not a concern. The potential impact of prevention rather than treatment after the fact would be great both on the health of infected persons and on the ability of those persons to transmit infection to others. The cost savings might be huge. Within a short few years, Shirley Ferebee Woolpert and her colleagues of the United States Public Health Service had organized a trial in nearly three thousand children in the United States. Further trials followed quickly, and by the end of the decade approximately thirty-five thousand Americans had taken isoniazid and a similar thirty-five thousand a placebo pill.[3]

The results were remarkable. One aspirin tablet-sized isoniazid pill each day—three hundred milligrams, approximately one one-hundredth of an ounce—prevented tuberculosis in all groups tested. Some types of persons were better protected than others. In general, those more recently infected and those of younger age benefitted the most. However, all were helped. Moreover, there were almost no side effects to this therapy. The pills were well tolerated; just as many placebo takers complained that the pill upset their stomachs as did isoniazid takers. There was no effect on mental function and none on pregnancy. Isoniazid appeared to be a true wonder drug.

The enormous size of the isoniazid trial renders it one of public health medicine's most exciting ventures ever. So also do some of the operating conditions. The Bethel region of western Alaska encompasses the drainage basin of the Kuskokwim and lower Yukon Rivers, nearly one hundred thousand square miles, a greater land area than that of eighty-five percent of all American states. At the time of the trial, most of the inhabitants lived in scattered villages, usually in small one room dwellings, subsisting on fishing and hunting. Their average income was less than three thousand dollars annually. Two percent of the residents of this area had active tuberculosis. Transportation was largely by boat and float plane in the summer, dog sled and ski plane in the winter. The field staff responsible for this vast project consisted of four nurses and a clerk. They enrolled and supervised more than seven thousand persons in the isoniazid prophylaxis study. The results in Bethel were as dramatic as they were elsewhere. Isoniazid prevented seventy percent of the expected cases of tuberculosis.[4]

The adage attributed to the mythical Murphy that if something can go wrong it most certainly will caught up with isoniazid prophylaxis for tuberculous infection in dramatic fashion in 1970. This form of preventive medicine had become widely accepted, and when two cafeteria workers in the United States Capitol Building were found to have tuberculosis, a tuberculin skin testing program was launched to identify all those at the Capitol Building infected by the tubercle bacillus and offer them isoniazid.[5] Much publicity was accorded this campaign, and many saw in it an opportunity to increase public awareness of tuberculosis in a dramatic fashion. Of course, many working in public health agencies also hoped that increased tax dollar funding for tuberculosis prevention campaigns would follow.

More than twenty-three hundred tuberculin skin test-positive Capitol Building workers began taking isoniazid. Within nine months, nineteen of them had developed liver disease, and two had died. One of those who died was the press secretary of a prominent congressman, and that resulted in a strident declamation on the floor of the House of Representatives. Among a similar number of uninfected employees who did not take the drug, only one case of liver disease occurred. The ensuing uproar was cacophonous. The rush to analyze the data by many experts produced no explanation other than that isoniazid taking was associated with the liver disease. Yet this complication had not been observed in the thirty-five thousand participants in the earlier trials. This discrepancy has never been completely explained, but it is now evident that isoniazid is capable of producing liver disease, albeit not at the rate once believed. If the drug is promptly discontinued, the liver disease resolves without further problems; if the drug is continued, death from liver failure may ensue.

It soon became apparent that the liver toxicity of isoniazid was related to daily alcohol use, to the concomitant use of certain uncommon medications, and to age. Age, in fact, proved to be the single most important factor that needed to be considered. In an elegant analysis, George Comstock, a distinguished Professor of Epidemiology at Johns Hopkins University, and Phyllis Edwards, Director of the Tuberculosis Control Division of the Centers for Disease Control, compared the competing risks of tuberculosis and isoniazid toxicity in relation to age.[6] While the liver disease risk increased with older age, the risk of tuberculosis in tuberculin reactors decreased with age, largely because persons previously infected outlived some of their risk with the passing of each year. They concluded that the risks were about equal at age forty-five. Subsequently, taking a somewhat conservative tack, American public health authorities recommended that isoniazid prophylaxis be used in persons less than thirty-five years old. With time, that recommendation has been modified to meet a number of special circumstances, but the basic concept of balancing risks has remained the guiding principal in the use of isoniazid prophylaxis. Thus qualified and administered with appropriate supervision, this form of preventive therapy has become one of the cornerstones of American tuberculosis public health policy.

Despite the acknowledged effectiveness of isoniazid prophylaxis and national endorsement of it as an important public health measure, we have been less than perfect in implementing its use. During 1991, American tuberculosis clinics reported nearly one hundred and twenty-seven thousand persons who were started on preventive treatment. Sixty-five percent of them completed the prescribed therapy; thirty-five percent did not.[7] That is, more than forty-four thousand Americans failed to comply with their doctor's recommendations.

Elsewhere in the world, the difficulties in mounting effective isoniazid prophylaxis campaigns have been greater, and this approach has met with rejection with a frequency equal to or greater than that in the United States. In high tuberculosis prevalence developing countries such programs have been uniformly unsuccessful. In fact, no country outside of North America has embraced this form of prevention as a part of its national tuberculosis control program.

It is an imperfect world. A simple, effective, safe, and cheap means of preventing tuberculosis, the number one killer among infectious diseases, the Captain of Death, has won only limited acceptance.

PART IV

Epilogue

You are the light of the world. A city set on a hill cannot be hid. Nor do men light a lamp and put it under a bushel, but on a stand, and it gives light to all in the house.

Let your light so shine before men, that they may see your good works. . . .

Matthew 4: 14–16[1]

26

Hope in Haiti

In 1961 James and Virginia Snavley visited Haiti on a vacation. Haiti was a romantic Caribbean vacation spot, notable not only for its balmy tropical climate and comfortable tourist hotels but also its vibrant culture. The African origins of its people were close to the surface, and mysterious voodoo traditions shaped the lives of Haitians. Haiti was both a popular and an exotic vacation destination. For the Snavleys, however, Haiti was something more. Haiti was a horror of need and poverty. Haiti was a call for help that they felt impelled to answer.

The following year, the Snavleys returned to Haiti, established residence in that country, and opened an orphanage. Their home for abandoned children was soon full, and they felt rewarded by their ability to care for these children. In 1965, they and some of their friends organized the Child Care Foundation to raise money in the United States to support the orphanage, and substantial contributions began to arrive, chiefly from protestant churches and their members. However, it soon became apparent to them that they had tackled a problem much too vast for their resources. The number of orphans needing shelter was much greater than they could ever hope to provide for, and there was little hope for placing those children whom they had succored. The Snavleys felt a need to redirect their efforts in a more sharply focused manner. After consultation with other missionaries, they decided to continue their work with children by opening a hospital for children with tuberculosis.

In December 1967, the Snavleys opened Grace Children's Hospital in Delmas, a newly developed area of Port-au-Prince where they had acquired the former home of the Mexican ambassador and land adjacent to it. Thirty seven children were admitted initially, but within a year the census had grown to seventy-five and the annual budget was fifty thousand dollars. Dr. Lyonel Théard, a Haitian pulmonary physician, was hired as medical director, and North American volunteers began arriving and providing needed administrative and nursing capability. The hospital was recognized by the Haitian government, and a franchise given to the hospital to permit duty-free importation of drugs to treat tuberculosis. Marie Bellande, a young, American-trained, Haitian nurse, who ultimately assumed a role of major administrative responsibility and leadership at Grace Children's Hospital and International Child Care, joined the hospital staff and then became its chief nurse. Additions were made to the hospital facility, and by 1974 the hospital had a census of two hundred children. Excellent care was given, although many of the very sick children admitted died before the drugs could control their disease. Children were usually hospitalized for one year before being discharged home, well.[2]

In 1974, the leaders of International Child Care made a major decision. Recognizing that treating two hundred children a year at Grace Children's Hospital would never have an important impact on Haiti's tuberculosis disease burden, the Child Care trustees committed themselves and their organization to take on tuberculosis treatment and control for the entire country. Let us examine the task they proposed to face.

Haiti, a crowded land of grinding poverty with no organized national health system, had at that time a population of about five million people, about one in ten of whom lived in Port-au-Prince, the capital city. Only three other communities exceeded twenty thousand. The population density was five hundred per square mile, similar to that of India and the highest in the Western Hemisphere. The per capita income was seventy dollars per year, the lowest in the hemisphere. Forty-two percent of the population was under the age of fourteen, reflecting the high birth rate, and fifty-seven percent of children died by age five. The country's medical services were provided chiefly by missionaries, and most Haitians simply had no medical care available to them. There was one doctor for every six thousand Haitians, and most of these professionals lived in Port-au-Prince. Rural Haitians were likely never to see a doctor in their lifetimes. The Minister of Health and his staff of one secretary had a small office in Port-au-Prince. The Bureau of Tuberculosis Control was housed in a dilapidated abandoned warehouse in the one corner still protected by a remaining portion of the original roof. There, the part-time director ran a small clinic for tuberculosis patients who could afford to pay. A government tuberculosis sanatorium in Port-au-Prince housed two hundred and thirty patients, and a similar number were sheltered in a former leprosarium southwest of the city; no treatment drugs were provided for the tuberculosis patients at the latter facility.[3]

Tuberculosis was thought to be the leading infectious disease problem in Haiti, although no figures were available to support this impression. Case report data collected by the Pan American Health Organization in the 1960s varied widely from year to year and provided little help in judging the extent of the problem Child Care faced. A number of isolated tuberculin skin test surveys had been made by various agencies in various regions of the country. They indicated that about ninety percent of adult Haitians were infected with tubercle bacilli and that about half of ten year old children were infected. From these limited data, we can judge that Child Care was about to face off in a fight against tuberculosis in Haiti with about two percent of the population—one hundred thousand people—needing treatment and with approximately one hundred and thirty persons being added to the sick roll each day. Of these numbers, about half were contagious to others, and the epidemic of tuberculosis in Haiti appeared to be in a stable balance, with the many new patients each day being matched by a similar number of deaths or spontaneous remissions. To win the fight, International Child Care would have to change that balance so that more of the sick became well and noncontagious and fewer of the well became sick.

The Croisade Anti Tuberculose was launched. The goals: vaccinate all children with BCG; find and treat every infectious case. And do these things in a country with few roads, none paved outside of Port-au-Prince. And in a country with no existing national health care system. And find the money to support this effort.

A mass BCG vaccination campaign was launched, organized and led by Henry Koop, an energetic, retired, Canadian pharmacist who moved to Haiti to volunteer his services. Mobile teams were organized. Traveling by Land Rover, by foot, by boat, or by mule, they covered the country. In each village, educational campaigns were mounted using local

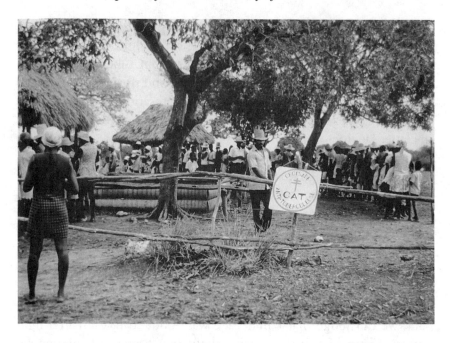

Figure 26.1. Line of persons waiting to receive BCG vaccination at a cock fight pit in Petit Trou de Nippes, Haiti in 1976. Photograph by the author.

community leaders and portable loudspeaker systems. Then, all children were vaccinated, the lines moving quickly past the automatic injector guns. In this fashion, eighty-five percent of rural Haitian children received BCG. In urban Port-au-Prince, the campaigns were somewhat less successful; urban dwellers are always harder to reach, especially in crowded slums.

Grace Children's Hospital underwent a dramatic transformation. Children were discharged after two or three months to continue their treatment in an ambulatory clinic. This made several wards available, and they were converted to clinic space. Soon, the clinic at Grace Children's Hospital was treating about four hundred children and a similar number of adults as ambulatory patients. While this change increased the number of tuberculosis victims who could be treated, that was not the primary reason for establishing and maintaining the clinic. Rather, the clinic and its supporting services were planned as a training center, a place where those who were to carry out a national case finding and treatment program could learn the necessary skills for diagnosing and treating tuberculosis.

As the vaccination teams moved across Haiti, they invited every mission, clinic, or health post they encountered to participate. Choose a case worker from your community, they challenged. Send that person to Grace Children's Hospital to be trained how to vaccinate children, how to make and interpret sputum smears, and how to give tuberculosis treatment. Then, Child Care promised, this local agent would return with a microscope, with supplies, and with medicines for treating tuberculosis. And as needed, these supplies would be renewed. Additionally, several physicians were recruited and trained to serve as expert supervisors, traveling day after day to support the growing network of tuberculosis agents working throughout the country. Within a decade, the program was treating about nine thousand patients each year countrywide.

Child Care's staff in Haiti grew to about two hundred. All but a very few were Haitian. Dr. Marie Renée Francisque, a Haitian physician with a Masters degree in Public Health from Johns Hopkins University, became the Medical Director. Money was needed, and Child Care's directors in the United States and Canada set about finding the funds to support a program with a budget that reached nearly two million dollars annually. Many churches from many denominations contributed as did even more individuals. The United Methodist Church made Child Care part of its denominationally-supported programs. Grants were obtained from foundations and from the United States Agency for International Development, the Canadian International Development Agency, and the World Bank. The troubled times of the 1980s and 1990s were particularly difficult, and during the international embargo imposed in an attempt to coerce Haiti into restoring elected President Aristide to power, Child Care's programs contracted, but continued.

A look at data collected at the Grace Children's Hospital Clinic during the 1980s and 1990s is revealing. In 1986 nearly thirty percent of patients failed to complete treatment for tuberculosis. Alarmed, the staff set out to change these figures. The clinic was reoriented to better serve the needs of its patients. Waiting time was reduced. Such ancillary services as family planning and nutrition were added. Mothers were given powdered milk as an incentive to attend. Staff members at all levels

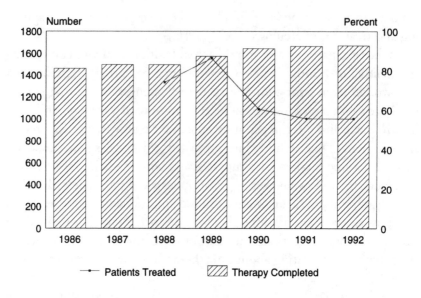

Figure 26.2. Number of patients treated and percent of patients completing treatment at Grace Children's Hospital in Port-au-Prince, Haiti for the period 1986 through 1992. Available data are incomplete with respect to the number of patients treated in 1986 and 1987. The remarkably high and improving percent of patients completing treatment resulted from an effort to make the clinic more responsive to the needs and wants of patients. Data from the annual reports of Grace Children's Hospital and from correspondence between the author and Dr. Marie Renée Francisque, Medical Director of International Child Care.

were taught to be more attentive to the needs of patients. These measures worked and, as seen in Figure 26.2, five years later ninety-three percent of patients successfully completed treatment. In contrast, at this time only eleven percent of patients discharged from Harlem Hospital in New York completed treatment (Chapter 6).

International Child Care's programs are not the only hopeful news from desperate Haiti. A program run jointly by the Centres pour Developpement et la Santé and Johns Hopkins University has treated tuberculosis patients in Cité Soleil, the worst of Port-au-Prince's slums. Of four hundred and twenty-seven patients who entered treatment between February 1990 and April 1992, of whom forty-two percent also had AIDS, more than eighty percent were cured. More than ninety percent adhered to their treatment regimens, and most of the deaths occurred among the patients who also had AIDS.[4]

In a rural treatment program in two villages in northern Haiti using only Haitian resources and not relying on help from other nations, three hundred and twenty-nine patients have been treated in a program under which the taking of drugs is directly observed to insure compliance. Seventy-nine percent were cured of their disease, twelve percent died, and only nine percent were lost to follow-up.[5]

It is, of course, important to ask whether the ambitious programs of International Child Care and others have changed the tuberculosis situation in Haiti. Certainly, care is now much more readily available to tuberculosis patients in Haiti. Human suffering has been relieved in thousands of persons. However, because of the long incubation period of tuberculosis, control measures in a country such as Haiti will have to be maintained for many decades before one can hope to see a real reduction in new cases of disease.

The important lesson to be learned from Haiti is that even under the most difficult situations of poverty and high disease prevalence, it is possible to implement measures for the control of tuberculosis and treatment of consumptive patients. In terms of the national annual budgets of most technologically advanced countries, the cost of attacking tuberculosis throughout the world is not high, but in terms of Haiti's resources, the costs are prohibitive. Should the world shoulder Haiti's problem? Regardless of one's humanitarian motives or lack of them, the answer to this question is yes. In the United States today more than one-third of all cases of tuberculosis occur in foreign born individuals. The Haitis of the world are the breeding grounds of our tuberculosis problem. It is a fallacy to think of tuberculosis in any but global terms. As we have seen, the history of tuberculosis is one of human triumph— triumph over the world's greatest killer. But the victory cannot be complete until the battle lines encircle the globe. No one is safe unti all are safe.

Hope in Haiti. Hope because Haiti demonstrates that dedicated people can vanquish the Captain of these Men of Death wherever it strikes.

Appendix I

Chronology

Chronology of events described in this book.

3000 BCE Earliest known portrayal of tuberculosis in Egyptian art.
2000   Reference to yakshma in India.
1000   Mummy of Egyptian girl. Peak of tuberculosis epidemic
          in Nile valley.
460   Birth of Hippocrates.
300   Reference to chiai nio in China.
          Medical school founded in Alexandria.
131 CE   Birth of Galen, who recommended milk for the treatment
          of tuberculosis.
496   Initiation of royal touch for scrofula by Clovis of France.
700   Mummy of Peruvian boy. Peak of tuberculosis epidemic
          in South and Central America.
1182   Birth of St. Francis.
1643   Death from tuberculosis of King Louis XIII of France.
1660   Sobriquet "Captain among these Men of Death" coined
          by Bunyan.
1677   Death from tuberculosis of Baruch Spinoza.
1680   Description of tubercles in lungs of consumptives by
          Franciscus Sylvius.
1699   Passage of Italian quarantine laws for tuberculosis.
1712   Samuel Johnson touched by Queen Anne for scrofula.
1720   Hypothesis that tuberculosis is caused by "animalcula" by
          Benjamin Martens.
1742   Horseback rides recommended by Thomas Sydenham for
          treatment of tuberculosis.

1796	William Jenner uses cowpox to perform the first vaccination for smallpox.
1815	Thomas Young estimates that one-fourth of European population is consumptive. Peak of tuberculosis epidemic in Europe.
1821	Death from tuberculosis of John Keats.
1826	Death from tuberculosis of René T.H. Laennec.
1831	Tuberculosis epidemic on Pitcairn Island.
1839	Frédéric Chopin and Georges Sand expelled from Mallorca.
1847	Death from tuberculosis of Marie Duplessis, model for Violetta in *La Traviata*.
1849	Death from tuberculosis of Frédéric Chopin.
1855	Death of Charlotte Brontë from tuberculosis.
1857	Channing Street shelter for tuberculosis patients opened in Boston by Harriet Ryan. Peak of tuberculosis epidemic in North America.
1859	Tuberculosis sanatorium, usually credited as the first such sanatorium, opened by Brehmer in Silesia.
1865	Demonstration of transmission of tuberculosis by Jean-Antoine Villemin.
1873	Arrival of Edward Livingston Trudeau in the Adirodacks.
1882	Discovery of the tubercle bacillus by Robert Koch.
1884	Adirondack Cottage Sanitarium opened at Saranac Lake by Trudeau.
1885	Louis Pasteur immunizes Joseph Meister against rabies. First thoracoplasty performed by De Cérenville.
1887-88	Sojourn at Saranac Lake of Robert Louis Stevenson.
1889	Promulgation of tuberculosis public health rules in New York City.
1890	Description of tuberculin by Robert Koch. Promulgation of tuberculin therapy for tuberculosis by Koch.
1892	Founding of first voluntary tuberculosis association in Philadelphia.
1894	First artificial pneumothorax induced by Forlanini.
1896	Premier of *La Bohème*.
1901	White Haven Sanatorium opened by Flick in Pennsylvania.

1902	Edmond Nocard isolates *M. bovis* strain used to develop BCG.
1904	Sale of first Christmas seal in Denmark.
1905	Robert Koch receives Nobel Prize.
1907	Clemens von Pirquet describes tuberculin skin test.
1912	Thomas Mann found to have tuberculosis while visiting his wife at Davos.
1921	First administration of BCG to a human.
1926	Max Lurie begins studies of tuberculosis in families of rabbits.
1930	Lübeck BCG catastrophe.
1934	Alice Marble collapses with tuberculosis.
1935-39	Aronson BCG trial.
1939	Publication of landmark cohort analysis by Wade Hampton Frost.
1941	Preparation of reference standard PPD by Florence Seibert.
	Demonstration of role of lymphocytes in tuberculous immunity by Merrill Chase.
1943	Josephine Baker develops tuberculosis.
	Discovery of Streptomycin by Selman Waksman.
1944	Patricia T. receives first injections of streptomycin.
1950	Death of George Orwell from tuberculosis.
1952	Recognition of T lymphocytes by Robert Good.
	Selman Waksman receives Nobel Prize.
	Sea View Hospital trial of isoniazid.
1954	Edith Lincoln suggests isoniazid prophylaxis.
	Adirondack Cottage Sanitarium in Saranac Lake closes.
1956	Recognition of B lymphocytes by Bruce Glick.
1957	Rifamycins isolated at Lepetit laboratories.
1959	Arden House Conference recommendations for elimination of tuberculosis.
1962	Death from tuberculosis of Eleanor Roosevelt.
1963	Demonstration of *in vitro* responses to PPD by Permain and colleagues and by Robert Schrek.
	Demonstration of immune granulomas by Kenneth Warren.

1967   Grace Children's Hospital opens in Haiti.
            Death of Vivien Leigh.
1970   Outbreak of isoniazid-related liver disease on Capitol Hill
            in Washington.
1973   World Health Organization endorsement of BCG.
1974   Croisade Antituberculose launched in Haiti.
1982   Publication of first description of AIDS.
1985   First national increase in tuberculosis case rate in the
            United States.
            Description of AIDS as Slim Disease in Uganda by David
            Serwadda and colleagues.
1986   Description of tuberculosis as a complication of AIDS by
            Gnana Sunderam, Lee Reichman, and colleagues.
1990   Appearance of Strain W multi drug-resistant tubercle
            bacilli in New York.

Appendix II

Glossary

Medical and Technical Terms Used in this Book

Acquired immunodeficiency syndrome. A disease of the human immune system caused by a virus and commonly known by its acronym, AIDS.

Actinomyces. A genus of microorganisms native to the soil that yielded many early antibiotics.

Actinomycete. A colloquial term for any one of the members of the genus *Actinomyces* and closely related organisms.

Active tuberculosis. Tuberculosis in its active state as defined by the presence of living tubercle bacilli or changing diseases process within the preceding six months.

AIDS. Acronym and common name for the acquired immunodeficiency syndrome.

Allergy. A state of altered reactivity to a precipitating agent, which is known as an antigen or allergen.

American Lung Association. Originally the National Association for the Study and Prevention of Tuberculosis, the oldest voluntary health agency, widely known for its Christmas seals.

American Thoracic Society. The largest American professional society of medical doctors specializing in pulmonary diseases. Originally the American Sanatorium Association and later the American Trudeau Society.

Antibiotic. A substance produced by a microorganism that is capable of arresting the growth of or killing other microorganisms.

Antibody. A protein in the blood serum that is induced by contact with and subsequently capable of reacting specifically with foreign substances, which are termed antigens.

Antigen. A foreign substance capable of inducing the formation of and reacting specifically with antibodies or sensitized lymphocytes.

Antiserum. Serum containing antibodies from the blood of a person or animal containing antibodies.

Arrested tuberculosis. Tuberculosis that no longer shows signs of activity—that is, is unchanging and no longer a source of living tubercle bacilli. Prior to the introduction of antibiotic therapy, tuberculosis was thought never to be cured, and the term arrested designated a currently healed state of disease that nevertheless was still thought to be capable of reactivating.

Artificial pneumothorax. A pneumothorax induced artificially by introducing air into the pleural cavity between the lung and the chest wall.

Attenuated. Literally, drawn out. This term is used to describe microorganisms that have become altered to be less virulent or non-virulent for humans.

Bacille Calmette-Guérin. An attenuated strain of *Mycobacterium bovis* developed by Calmette and Guérin as a vaccine against tuberculosis. Commonly known by its acronym, BCG.

Bacillus. This term is commonly used generically to describe microorganisms and as a synonym for bacterium. More narrowly defined, it refers specifically to members of the genus *Bacillus*, long, thin bacteria with specific growth, reproductive, and staining characteristics.

Bactericidal. An adjective used to describe drugs capable of killing bacteria.

Bacteriostatic. An adjective used to describe drugs capable of halting the growth of but not killing bacteria.

Bacterium. A term commonly used to designated a type of single-celled microorganism, including many that produce disease.

B-cell. A colloquial designation for B-lymphocyte.

BCG. The acronym and colloquial term for Bacille Calmette-Guérin, a vaccine against tuberculosis.

B-lymphocyte. A class of lymphocyte specialized for the production of antibody.

Bronchus. A tubular airway, a series of which connect the trachea (wind pipe) with the lungs.

Bursa of Fabricius. A specialized organ of the hind gut of the chicken associated with the production of B-lymphocytes in these birds. The term B-lymphocyte derives from this association.

Cavity. A hole or vacant space within an area of diseased tissue and a result of the disease process. Similar to an abscess, but usually used in conjunction with processes such as tuberculosis that are more chronic in nature than diseases associated with abscesses.

CD4⁺ T-lymphocyte. A subclass of T-lymphocytes responsible for immunologic memory and promoting cellular immune responses. These cells are recognizable by surface antigens that can be identified with appropriate antisera.

Chemotherapy. The treatment of disease with chemical agents. While this term is most commonly known today as a form of cancer treatment, the term is also applied to the treatment of tuberculosis with drugs.

Cohort. An epidemiological term used to designate a group of individuals sharing one or more defining common characteristics.

Consumption. An older term for tuberculosis.

Cytokine. A substance produced by one cell and capable of reacting with and inducing responses in other cells of the same or different types. This term is usually reserved for substances and cells of the immune system.

Delayed hypersensitivity. A type of immune response mediated by specific lymphocytes and characterized by an onset delayed by one or two days after reexposure to the inciting antigen. This type of hypersensitivity is characteristic of tuberculosis.

Desensitization. The process of rendering an allergic individual no longer responsive to an antigen by repeated exposure to the antigen under certain conditions.

DNA. The acronym and colloquial name for deoxyribonucleic acid. Genes are composed of specific configurations of this complex molecule.

Endotoxin. A substance in the cell wall of certain bacteria that causes local pain, fever, and shock in humans and animals.

Epidemic. Literally, upon a people. An outbreak of disease in a population.

Epidemiologist. A scientist trained to study epidemics.

Epidemiology. The science of the study of epidemics.

Ethambutol. A bacteriostatic drug used for treatment of tuberculosis.

Extrapleural plombage. A surgical procedure in which material is placed between the ribs and the pleura lining the chest cavity so as to occupy space within the chest and compress the underlying lung. The procedure was used as a means of collapse therapy for tuberculosis.

Fomes, fomites (plural). Strictly defined, any inanimate object or particle capable of transmitting infection by absorbing germs onto and transmitting them from its surface. Generally used to refer to sedentary particles rather than air-born particles.

Genus. A taxonomic term used to designate a group of related species of organisms.

Gramicidin. An antibiotic isolated by René Dubos and used for topical treatment of wound infections.

Granuloma. An immunologically-mediated tissue inflammatory response typical of delayed hypersensitivity reactions. The characteristic tissue response to tuberculosis.

Hemoptysis. The coughing of blood.

HIV. An acronym for human immunodeficiency virus.

Human immunodeficiency virus. The virus that causes the acquired immunodeficiency syndrome (AIDS).

Hypersensitivity. An altered state of reactivity with increased responses. This term is typically applied to allergic responses.

Immune. Classically, this term means resistant to infection or disease. In modern usage, this term is often limited to the case where the resistance is acquired and is mediated by specific, antigen-induced, lymphocyte or antibody-mediated host responses.

Immunity. The state or condition of being immune.

Immunodeficiency. A lack of immunity under circumstances where immunity would ordinarily exist.

Immunologist. A scientist trained to study immunity.

Immunology. The science of the study of immunity.

Inactive tuberculosis. Tuberculosis showing no current signs of activity.

Incidence. The rate of occurrence of a disease or a condition within a specified period of time. Often expressed for tuberculosis as the number of new cases per one hundred thousand population per year.

Infection. The acquisition of a germ capable of producing disease. Infection with *M. tuberculosis* does not always lead to disease.

INH. Commonly used abbreviation and short name for isoniazid.

Iproniazid. Isomer of isoniazid, also known as marsilid.

Isoniazid. Isonicotinic acid hydrazide. A bactericidal drug used for the treatment of tuberculosis.

Lupus vulgaris. Tuberculosis of the skin. An archaic dermatologic term not commonly used today.

Lymphocyte. The class of white blood cells that includes cells with immunologic functions, including immunologic memory.

Lymphokine. A cytokine produced by lymphocytes.

M. avium. Shortened form of *Mycobacterium avium.*

M. bovis. Shortened form of *Mycobacterium bovis.*

M. tuberculosis. Shortened form of *Mycobacterium tuberculosis.*

Macrophage. A large white blood cell and tissue cell capable of ingesting materials and particles foreign to the host. This cell participates in cellular (delayed) immune responses. It is the principal cell present in granulomas. When circulating in the blood, it is usually known as a monocyte.

Microbe. A bacterium or germ. A microorganism.

Microbiologist. A scientist trained in the study of microorganisms.

Microbiology. The science of the study of microorganisms.

Microorganism. An organism or life form too small to be seen without the aid of a microscope, such as a microbe.

Miliary tuberculosis. Tuberculosis that has spread through the blood stream to seed all organs of the body. The term miliary originated with early pathologists performing autopsies on tuberculosis patients who noted that the small granulomas or tubercles in the lungs looked like millet seeds.

Monocyte. A large white blood cell that enters tissues to participate in immune responses. In tissues it is known as a macrophage.

Mycobacterium. The genus of bacteria that includes the tubercle bacillus and related species. By convention, genus names are always written out when first used in a text and capitalized but thereafter may be abbreviated with the first letter only followed by a period (*M.*).

Mycobacterium avium. An environmental, soil and water species of *Mycobacterium* that is usually not pathogenic for immunologically normal humans but frequently produces disseminated disease in persons with AIDS. The nomenclature originated because this organism was first isolated from a chicken.

Mycobacterium bovis. The bovine type of tubercle bacillus. It causes disease in cattle and also in many other mammals including humans.

Mycobacterium tuberculosis. The scientific name for the tubercle bacillus. The bacterium that causes tuberculosis.

National Tuberculosis Association. A voluntary health agency devoted to fighting tuberculosis. Name changed and later became the American Lung Association.

Old tuberculin. Tuberculin. Termed old tuberculin because old liquid cultures are used for preparation. All tuberculin in use for tuberculin tests today is old tuberculin.

OT. Colloquial designation for old tuberculin.

Pathogenesis. The evolution of a disease process as related to its cause.

Para-aminosalicylic acid. Bacteriostatic drug used for treating tuberculosis.

PAS. Para-aminosalicylic acid.

Penicillin. An antibiotic in widespread use for treating many infections. Not active against tubercle bacilli.

Phlebotomy. Puncture of a vein, usually for the purpose of withdrawing blood.

Phrenic nerve. The nerve that innervates the diaphragm. The right and left phrenic nerves leave the spinal cord high in the neck and pass through the neck and chest cavity to reach the diaphragm.

Phthisis. The ancient Greek word for tuberculosis. It remained in use in medical terminology well through the nineteenth century.

Plasma. The liquid phase of unclotted blood.

Placebo. An inactive and harmless medicine often given to control subjects in a clinical drug trial so that neither the trial subjects nor the evaluators will know which subjects are receiving the drug being studied.

Pleura. The membrane lining the chest cavity and covering the surfaces of the lungs.

Pleurisy. Inflammation of the pleura.

Pleurisy with effusion. Pleurisy accompanied by the accumulation of fluid in the pleural space. A common manifestation of tuberculosis, especially primary tuberculosis.

Plombage. Extrapleural plombage. The introduction of material between the pleura and the ribs to reduce the size of the chest cavity and collapse the underlying lung. A surgical procedure used for the treatment of tuberculosis, especially in attempts to close cavities.

Pneumoperitoneum. The presence of air in the abdominal cavity. The introduction of air into the abdominal cavity so as to elevate the diaphragm and cause collapse of the lung. A procedure used for the treatment of tuberculosis, especially in attempts to close cavities.

Pneumothorax. The presence of air in the pleural space. The introduction of air into the pleural cavity between the lung and the chest wall so as to cause collapse of the lung. A procedure used for the treatment of tuberculosis, especially in attempts to close cavities.

PPD. Purified protein derivative of tuberculin.

Prevalence. The amount of disease present in a population at any given time usually expressed as a ratio, fraction, or percent, often for tuberculosis as the number of cases per one hundred thousand.

Primary tuberculosis. Tuberculosis occurring directly following initial infection with tubercle bacilli. The first tuberculosis disease episode. Often a mild and unnoticed illness with spontaneous remission.

Prophylaxis. Disease prevention, preventive treatment.

Prontosil. A red dye found to be bacteriostatic for many bacteria. Its active moiety was sulfanilamide, the first sulfonamide drug.

Purified protein derivative. A material prepared from tuberculin that is semipurified and more readily standardized than crude tuberculin. Commonly known by its acronym, PPD, and the material commonly used for tuberculin testing today.

Radiograph. An image made by passing Xrays through opaque objects such as the human body.

Radiologist. A doctor trained in radiology.

Radiology. The science of and branch of medicine devoted to making and studying images made by passing Xrays through opaque objects such as the human body.

Respiration. The metabolic life process that consumes oxygen and produces carbon dioxide. Also, the act of breathing during which oxygen is absorbed and carbon dioxide excreted.

Respiratory. An adjective used to describe a process or processes related to respiration.

Rifamycin. An antibiotic derived from *Streptomyces mediterranei.*

Rifampicin. Rifampin.

Rifampin. An antibiotic synthesized from rifamycin that is bactericidal for tubercle bacilli.

Roentgenogram. An image made by passing Xrays through opaque objects such as the human body. A radiograph. The term honors William Roentgen, the discoverer of Xrays and the person who first used Xrays for imaging.

Roentgenograph. A roentgenogram.

Roentgenology. Radiology.

Sanatorium. A hospital or health facility providing treatment for chronic disease, especially tuberculosis. Sometimes used synonymously with sanitarium. Sanatorium is used throughout this book, except in referring to the Adirondack Cottage Sanitarium, founded by Trudeau and named thus by him.

Sanitarium. A term often used synonymously with sanatorium. Originally, sanitarium meant a spa or facility for general health promotion, but not an institution for specific treatment of diseases.

Scrofula. Tuberculosis of the lymph nodes in the neck. The term derives from a Latin word meaning little pig or suckling sow. The swelling produced in the neck was said to cause children with scrofula to have a neck like that of a pig.

Serum. The liquid phase of clotted blood. Sometimes used synonymously with antiserum.

Species. A taxonomic group of organisms sufficiently closely related so as to be considered of a single type. By convention, species names are not abbreviated, are not capitalized, and are italicized.

Spores. The reproductive units of some microbes, analogous to seeds of plants. Spores are usually hardy and resist most extremes of environmental conditions.

Sputum. Respiratory secretions, especially expectorated secretions.

Streptomyces griseus. The soil microbe from which streptomycin was isolated.

Streptomyces mediterranei. The soil microbe from which rifamycin was isolated.

Streptomycin. An antibiotic isolated from *Streptomyces griseus* by Selman Waksman and Albert Schatz. It is bactericidal for tubercle bacilli.

Sulfonamide. One of a group of closely related drugs effective in treating many infections. Not useful for the treatment of tuberculosis.

TB. Colloquial term for tuberculosis.

T-cell. A colloquial designation for T-lymphocyte.

Thiacetazone. Thioacetazone.

Thioacetazone. A semithiocarbazone drug that is bacteriostatic against tubercle bacilli. Not used in the United States. Widely used in developing countries because of its low cost.

Thoracoplasty. A surgical procedure designed to collapse diseased lung by removal of portions of ribs to reshape the chest wall.

Thymus. A gland located in the neck that is important during neonatal life in the differentiation of T-lymphocytes.

T-lymphocyte. A lymphocyte named for its relation to the thymus gland and responsible for immunologic memory and mediation of delayed hypersensitivity reactions.

Trachea. The central windpipe. The airway beginning at the larynx and connecting the mouth and nose with bronchi leading to the lungs.

Tubercle. A granuloma due to tuberculosis.

Tubercle bacillus. A colloquial term for *Mycobacterium tuberculosis*, the microbe that causes tuberculosis.

Tubercular. Strictly defined, an adjective meaning having tubercles. Commonly, and in a strict sense incorrectly, used as a synonym for tuberculous.

Tuberculin. The sterile filtrate of liquid cultures of tubercle bacilli. It contains many antigens of tubercle bacilli and is injected in small quantities as a diagnostic aid for identifying individuals infected with tubercle bacilli.

Tuberculin purified protein derivative. Purified protein derivative, PPD.

Tuberculin skin test. Tuberculin test.

Tuberculin test. A test in which a small amount of dilute tuberculin or PPD is introduced into the skin. A reaction to the introduced antigen is termed a positive tuberculin test and indicates prior infection with the tubercle bacillus.

Tuberculosis. The chronic, wasting disease caused by *Mycobacterium tuberculosis* or *M. bovis*.

Tuberculous. An adjective meaning having tuberculosis or related to tuberculosis.

Virulence. The capacity of a microorganism to produce disease.

Virulent. Possessing virulence.

Xray. A form of radiation capable of passing through opaque objects such as the human body and used for making radiographs. Often used mistakenly in colloquial speech as a synonym for radiograph.

Notes

Introduction

1. Bunyan J. The life and death of Mr. Badman. New York: R.H. Russell, 1900.
2. Dolin PJ, Raviglione MC, Kochi A. Global tuberculosis incidence and mortality. Bull World Health Org 1994; 72:213-20. Raviglione MC, Snider DE Jr, Kochi, A. Global epidemiology of tuberculosis. Morbidity and mortality of a worldwide epidemic. JAMA 1995; 273:220-6. These two papers are from the Tuberculosis Program of the World Health Organization.

Chapter 1: An Egyptian Girl; A Peruvian Boy

1. Deuteronomy 28:22. The Holy Bible. Revised standard version. New York: Thomas Nelson and Sons, 1953.
2. Zimmerman MR. Pulmonary and osseous tuberculosis in an Egyptian mummy. Bull NY Acad Med 1979; 55:604-8. . This account of a prehistoric Egyptian girl is based on the detailed study of a mummy by Zimmerman. The sex of the mummified child is not identified by Zimmerman; I have chosen to tell the story of a little girl.
3. Cave AJE. The evidence for the incidence of tuberculosis in ancient Egypt. Brit J Tuberc 1939; 33:142-52. The mummy of Nesperehân is among the most carefully studied of all Egyptian mummies and the evidence for tuberculosis is clear. In his paper, Professor Cave also provides interesting information on the representation of spinal tuberculosis in early Egyptian art. Morse D, Brothwell DR, Ucko PJ. Tuberculosis in ancient Egypt. Am Rev Respir Dis 1964; 90:524-41. This later

and often cited study of early Egyptian tuberculosis relies heavily on the descriptions of Cave.

4. Allison MJ, Mendoza D, Pezzia A. Documentation of a case of tuberculosis in pre-Columbian America. Am Rev Respir Dis 1973; 107:985-91. Marvin Allison and his Peruvian colleagues have contributed greatly to our knowledge of prehistoric diseases of the Andean region. The crippled Peruvian child was described in detail by them.

5. Salo W, Aufderheide AC, Buikstra J, Holcomb TA. Identification of *Mycobacterium tuberculosis* DNA in a pre-Columbian Peruvian mummy. Proc Natl Acad Sci USA 1994; 91:2091-4. This investigation confirms the earlier identification by staining and microscopic examination of tubercle bacilli in Peruvian mummies. It further limits the identification to a group of bacilli known collectively as the *Mycobacterium tuberculosis* complex, including *M. tuberculosis* and *M. bovis*. It excludes the always unlikely possibility that the earlier identification was of related soil or water organisms.

6. Ponce Sanginés C. Tenupa y Ekaku. La Paz, Bolivia: Los Amigos del Libro, 1969. Dr. Ponce, who served as the Secretary of the Bolivian National Academy of Sciences, spent many years as curator of the Tiwanaku archaeological site in Bolivia.

7. Daniel TM. An immunochemist's view of the epidemiology of tuberculosis. In: Buikstra JE, editor. Prehistoric tuberculosis in the Americas. Evanston, IL: Northwestern University Archaeologic Program, 1981:35-48. The symposium volume edited by Buikstra in which this paper is published contains other papers of relevance to the prehistoric occurrence of tuberculosis in the central plains of North America. Black FS. Infectious diseases in primitive societies. Science 1975; 1187:515-8. This paper provides further data relevant to the prevalence of tuberculous infection among primitive peoples of the Amazon basin.

8. Thomas H. Conquest. Montezuma, Cortés, and the fall of old Mexico. New York: Simon and Schuster, 1993:26.

9. Arriaza BT, Salo W, Aufderheide AC, Holcomb TA. Pre-Columbian tuberculosis in northern Chile: Molecular and skeletal evidence. Am J Phys Anthropol 1995; 98:37-45.

10. Brown L. The story of clinical pulmonary tuberculosis. Baltimore: The Williams & Wilkins Company, 1941:3.

11. Gibbons A. The peopling of the Americas. Science 1996; 274:31-3.

12. Manchester K. Tuberculosis and leprosy in antiquity: An interpretation. Med Hist 1984; 28:162-73. Bates JH, Stead WW. The history of tuberculosis as a global epidemic. Med Clin N Amer 1993; 77:1205-17. Haas F, Haas SS. The origins of *Mycobacterium tuberculosis* and the notion of its contagiousness. In: Rom WN, Garay S, editors. Tuberculosis. Boston: Little, Brown, and Company, 1996:3-19. The view that *Mycobacterium bovis* caused most prehistoric tuberculosis and that *M. tuberculosis* evolved from its cattle-infecting cousin at a fairly recent date was widely espoused by medical historians prior to the conclusive demonstration of tuberculosis in pre-Columbian South American mummies. As noted in the text, this view is difficult to sustain today.

13. McGrath JW. Social networks of disease spread in the lower Illinois valley: A simulation approach. Am J Phys Anthro 1988; 77:483-96.

14. Daniel, TM. Op cit.

Chapter 2: Kos, Alexandria, and Rome

1. Meachen GN. A short history of tuberculosis. London: Staples Press Limited, 1936.

2. Leviticus 26:16. The Holy Bible. Revised Standard Version. New York: Thomas Nelson and Sons, 1953. Deuteronomy 28:22. Op cit.

3. Hippocrates. Book I. Of the Epidemics. The text quoted is from Major RH. Classic descriptions of disease. With biographical sketches of the authors. Third edition. Springfield, IL: Charles C. Thomas, 1945:52-53.

4. Guthrie D. A history of medicine. Philadelphia: J. B. Lippincott, 1946. Among many texts of medical history dealing with classic times, this one is readable and contains much information relevant to the material on tuberculosis presented here.

5. Gordon BL. Medieval and renaissance medicine. New York: Philosophical Library, 1959:476.

Chapter 3: The Middle Ages and Beyond

1. Locy WA, 1908. Cited by Myers JA. Captain of all these men of

death. Tuberculosis historical highlights. St. Louis: Warren H. Green, 1977:16.

2. Krause AK. Tuberculosis and public health. Am Rev Tuberc 1928; 18:271-322. Long ER. The decline of tuberculosis with special reference to its generalized form. Bull Hist Med 1940; 8:819-43. Meaningful estimates of the prevalence of tuberculosis in Europe during the dark ages are difficult to find. I have relied heavily upon the estimates of Krause and, to a lesser extent, of Long.

3. Garrison FH. An Introduction to the history of medicine, Fourth edition. Philadelphia: W.B. Saunders Co., 1929:245-309. Guthrie D. A history of medicine. Philadelphia: J.B. Lippincott Company, 1946: 176-214. Gordon BL. Medieval and renaissance medicine. New York: Philosophical Library, 1959:474-80. Excellent descriptions of the King's Evil and the use of the royal touch for its cure are provided in several texts of medical history. I have relied chiefly on the three cited above; two others are listed below: Crawford R. The king's evil. Oxford: Oxford Press, 1911. An informative book on this subject. Bloch M (translated by Anderson JE). The royal touch. Sacred monarchy and scrofula in England and France. Montreal: McGill-Queen's University Press, 1973. A book of somewhat broader scope with much relevant material.

4. Clifford JL. Young Sam Johnson. New York: McGraw-Hill Book Company, 1955.

5. Moorman L.J. Tuberculosis and genius. Chicago: The University of Chicago Press, 1940: 259-67.

6. Browne L. Blesséd Spinoza. A biography of the philosopher. New York: The MacMillan Company, 1932.

7. Myers JA. Captain of all these men of death. Tuberculosis historical highlights. St. Louis: Warren H. Green, 1977.

8. Krause AK. Op cit.

9. Bunyan J. The life and death of Mr. Badman. New York: R.H. Russell, 1900.

Chapter 4: The Relentless Tide

1. McNeill WH. Plagues and peoples. New York: Doubleday, 1977. Although tuberculosis is not accorded major note, McNeill presents an

interesting discussion of the transglobal sweep of many infectious diseases. Krause RM. The restless tide: The persistent challenge of the microbial world. Washington: National Foundation for Infectious Diseases, 1981. The inevitable resurgence of infectious diseases is discussed
by the distinguished infectious disease specialist Richard M. Krause.
This discussion by Krause focuses on the ability of microorganisms to
succeed despite medicine's interventions.

    2. The first infectious disease to be eradicated from the earth was
small-pox. Poliomyelitis has now been eradicated from the Americas,
and global eradication will soon follow. Measles will almost certainly be
the next to disappear. Vaccination has been the key instrument in achieving these victories. Daniel TM, Robbins FC. Polio. Rochester, NY: The
University of Rochester Press, 1997.

    3. Morton R. Cited by Myers JA. Captain of all these men of death.
Tuberculosis historical highlights. St. Louis: Warren H. Green, 1977:23.

    4. Long ER. The decline of tuberculosis with special reference to its
generalized form. Bull Hist Med 1940; 8:819-43.

    5. Gallagher R. Diseases that plague modern man. A history of ten
communicable diseases. Chapter 11. Tuberculosis. Dobbs Ferry, NY:
Oceana Publications, 1969:167-78.

    6. Scannell JG. A world of wonders. Harvard Medical Alumni Bul-
letin 1992(Summer):24-25. The author erroneously identified the skeletal deformity depicted as kyphoscoliosis. Daniel TM. Diagnosis disputed (letter). Harvard Medical Alumni Bulletin 1992(Autumn):3. The
mistaken identification by Scannel was corrected in this letter to the
editor.

    7. Fraser R. The Brontës. Charlotte Brontë and her family. New
York: Crown Publishers, 1988. There have been many volumes recount-
ing the lives of the Brontës. I have relied chiefly on Fraser's book.

    8. Ibid:319.

    9. Koch R. Die aetiologie der tuberculose, a translation by Berna
Pinner and Max Pinner with an introduction by Allen K. Krause. Am
Rev Tuberc 1932; 25:285-323. Koch's estimates are credible, for he was
certainly the greatest observer of tuberculosis of his time. For more about
this extraordinary scientist and physician, see Chapter 8. Krause, who
translated this article, was an associate of E.L. Trudeau, who was among
the first to repeat and verify Koch's studies in America.

10. Richman M. The man who made John Harvard. Harvard Magazine 1977; 80:46-51.

11. Metropolitan opera libretto. La traviata. New York: Fred Rullman, 1950.

12. Libretto. La bohème. Radio Corporation of America, 1952.

13. Holmberg SD. The rise of tuberculosis in America before 1820. Am Rev Respir Dis 1990; 142:1228-32. This excellent scholarly paper is well referenced and cites many primary sources of great interest.

14. Perzigian AJ, Widmer L. Evidence for tuberculosis in a prehistoric population. JAMA 1979; 241:2643-46.

15. Pfeiffer S. Paleopathology in an Iroquoian ossuary, with special reference to tuberculosis. Am J Phys Anthropol 1984; 65:181-9.

16. Paulsen HJ. Tuberculosis in the Native American: Indigenous or introduced? Rev Infect Dis 1987; 9:1180-6.

17. Comstock GW, Philip RN. Decline of the tuberculosis epidemic in Alaska. Publ Hlth Rep 1961; 76:19-24. Grzybowski S, Styblo K, Dorken E. Tuberculosis in Eskimos. Tubercle 1976; 57(suppl):S1-S58.

18. Wilkinson E. Notes of the prevalence of tuberculosis in India. Proc Royal Soc Med 1914; 8:195-225.

19. Shapiro HL. The heritage of the Bounty; The story of Pitcairn through six generations. New York: Simon and Schuster, 1936. Silverman D. Pitcairn Island. Cleveland: World Publishing Company, 1967. While the story of the Bounty mutiny is well known, the fate of the mutineers and their descendants is less familiar. Easily readable scholarly accounts are provided by the two sources cited.

20. Robertson HE. Quoted in Grigg ERN. The arcana of tuberculosis. With a brief epidemiologic history of the disease in the U.S.A. Am Rev Tuberc Pulm Dis 1958; 78:151-72.

21. McKeown T. Medicine and world population. J Chron Dis 1965; 18:1067-77. McKeown T. The origins of human disease. Oxford: Basil Blackwell, 1988. In this book McKeown summarizes and develops more fully his theses presented in earlier publications.

22. McKeown T. A historical appraisal of the medical task. In: McLachlan G, McKeown T, editors. Medical history and medical care. A symposium of perspectives. London: Oxford University Press, 1971:29-55.

23. Edwards LB, Livesay VT, Acquaviva FA, Palmer CE. Height,

weight, tuberculous infection, and tuberculous disease. Arch Environ Hlth 1971; 22:106-12.

24. Wilson LG. The historical decline of tuberculosis in Europe and America: Its causes and significance. J Hist Med Allied Sc 1990; 45:366-96.

25. Davis AL. History of the sanitorium movement. In: Rom WN, Garay SM. Tuberculosis. Boston: Little, Brown and Company, 1996:35-54. Dr. Davis' account is well researched and highly readable. She has a great interest in the subject and served as the medical director of the tuberculosis service at Bellvue Hopsital in New York for many years.

26. Devadatta S, Dawson JJY, Fox W, Janardhanam B, et al. Attack rate of tuberculosis in a 5-year period among close family contacts of tuberculosis patients under domiciliary treatment with isoniazid plus PAS or isoniazid alone. Bull Wld Hlth Org 1970; 42:337-351.

27. Grigg ERN. The arcana of tuberculosis. With a brief epidemiologic history of the disease in the U.S.A. Am Rev Tuberc Pulm Dis 1958; 78:151-72.

28. Bates JH, Stead WW. The history of tuberculosis as a global epidemic. Med Clin N Amer 1993; 77:1205-17. Stead WW, Eisenach KD, Cave MD, Beggs ML, et al. When did Mycobacterium tuberculosis infection first occur in the New World? An important question with public health implications. Am J Resp Crit Care Med 1995; 151:1267-8.

29. Mitchell A. An inexact science: The statistics of tuberculosis in late nineteenth-century France. The Society for the Social History of Medicine 1990:387-403.

Chapter 5: The Hope for Eradication

1. Feldberg GD. Disease and class. Tuberculosis and the shaping of modern North American society. New Brunswick, NJ: Rutgers University Press, 1995:5,117-18. Eleanor Roosevelt's illness is not well documented, and conflicting descriptions occur in the several biographies I consulted. Feldberg provides the most credible and well documented account of her early disease. However, on the basis of my reading of Roosevelt's biographies and conversations with physicians I believe to

have been conversant with her illness, I have placed her pleurisy at a somewhat earlier age than implied by Feldberg. Lash JP. A world of love. Eleanor Roosevelt and her friends. 1943-1962. Garden City, NY: Doubleday and Company, 1984. Lash provides the most credible description of Roosevelt's terminal illness. It provides quotes from her attending physician. Some accounts of Roosevelt's illness strike the modern, medically-oriented reader as intended to deceive the public, perhaps reminiscent of her husband's earlier deceptions with respect to his paralysis from poliomyelitis.

2. Maxcy KF. Papers of Wade Hampton Frost, M.D. A contribution to epidemiological method. New York: The Commonwealth Fund, 1941.

3. Grigg ERN. The arcana of tuberculosis. With a brief epidemiologic history of the disease in the U.S.A. Part III. Epidemiologic history of tuberculosis in the United States. Am Rev Tuberc Pulm Dis 1958; 78:426-53. This paper not only provides extensive data on the epidemiology of tuberculosis in the United States in the nineteenth and early twentieth centuries, but it also provides information on prominent historical figures who were afflicted by the disease.

4. Frost WH. The age selection of mortality from tuberculosis in successive decades. Am J Hyg 1939; 30:91-6.

5. Cited by Comstock GW. Advances toward the conquest of tuberculosis. Publ Hlth Rep 1980; 95:444-50.

6. Styblo K, Meijer J. Recent advances in tuberculosis epidemiology with regard to formulation or re-adjustment of control programmes. Bull Internat Union Against Tuberc 1978; 53:283-94.

7. Lowell AM. Tuberculosis in the world. Trends in tuberculosis incidence, prevalence, and mortality at the beginning of the 3rd decade of the chemotherapeutic era. Atlanta, GA: US Department of Health, Education, and Welfare, Public Health Service Center for Disease Control (HEW Publication No. CDC 76-8317), 1976.

8. American Lung Association Bulletin, October 1981:13-5. American Thoracic Society News, October 1987:3-4.

9. American Lung Association Bulletin, March 1982:11-3. Haygood TM. Radiologic history exhibit. Chest screening and tuberculosis in the United States. RadioGraphics 1994; 14:1151-66.

10. The photograph is from the American Lung Association publica-

tion cited. The biographical information is based on my personal communication with the girl's parents.

11. Comstock GW. The international tuberculosis campaign: A pioneering venture in mass vaccination and research. Clin Infect Dis 1994; 19:528-40. The story of this effort is recounted in delightful, anecdotal style by Comstock. I personally recall a delightful conversation with Dr. Holm in 1971, during which he emphasized that if one waited to be asked to mount a relief mission, the relief would never arrive in a timely fashion.

12. Ochs CW. The epidemiology of tuberculosis. JAMA 1962; 179:247-52.

13. The Arden House conference on tuberculosis. US Department of Health Education and Welfare, Public Health Service Publication No. 784, 1960.

14. Centers for Disease Control. A strategic plan for the elimination of tuberculosis in the United States. Morbidity and Mortality Weekly Report 1989; 38(S-3):1-25.

Chapter 6: The Failed Conquest

1. Sunderam G, McDonald RJ, Maniatis T, Oleske J, Kapila R, Reichman LB. Tuberculosis as a manifestation of the acquired immunodeficiency syndrome (AIDS). JAMA 1986; 256:362-6.

2. Selwyn PA, Hartel D, Lewis VA, Schoenbaum EE, et al. A prospective study of the risk of tuberculosis among intravenous drug users with human immunodeficiency virus infection. New Engl J Med 1989; 320:545-50.

3. Di Perri G, Cruciani M, Danzi MC, Luzatti R, et al. Nosocomial epidemic of active tuberculosis among HIV-infected patients. Lancet 1989; 2:1502-4.

4. Daley CL, Small PM, Schecter GF, Schoolnik GK, et al. An outbreak of tuberculosis with accelerated progression among persons infected with the human immunodeficiency virus. N Engl J Med 1992; 326:231-5.

5. Brudney K, Dobkin J. Resurgent tuberculosis in New York City.

Human immunodeficiency virus, homelessness, and the decline of tuberculosis control programs. Am Rev Respir Dis 1991; 144:745-9.

6. Allen C, Berg J, Blatt L, Foster V, Furlong J, Schade CP. INH-resistant tuberculosis in an urban high school—Oregon. MMWR 1980; 29:194-6.

7. Hermans PWM, Messadi F, Guebrexabher F, van Soolingen D, et al. Analysis of the population structure of *Mycobacterium tuberculosis* in Ethiopia, Tunisia, and the Netherlands: Usefulness of DNA typing for global tuberculosis epidemiology. J Infect Dis 1995; 171:1504-13.

8. Centers for Disease Control. 1987 tuberculosis statistics in the United States. Atlanta: U.S. Department of Health and Human Services, 1989. HHS Publication No. (CDC) 89-8322.

9. Tuberculosis Programme. Tuberculosis notification update July 1992. Geneva: World Health Organization, 1992.

10. Frieden TR, Sterling T, Pablos-Mendez A, Kilburn JO, Cauthen GM, Dooley SW. The emergence of drug-resistant tuberculosis in New York City. New Engl J Med 1993; 328:521-6.

11. Ibid.

12. Bifani PJ, Plikaytis BB, Kapur V, Stockbauer K, et al. Origin and interstate spread of a New York City multidrug-resistant *Mycobacterium tuberculosis* clone family: Adverse implications for tuberculosis control in the 21st century. JAMA 1996; 275:452-7. Additional information concerning strain W comes from my personal records concerning the Ohio patient, for whom I provided medical care.

13. Reichman LB. The U-shaped curve of concern. Am Rev Respir Dis 1991; 144:741-742.

14. Brudney K, Dobkin J. A tale of two cities: Tuberculosis control in Nicaragua and New York City. Seminars Resp Infect 1991; 6:261-272.

15. Division of Tuberculosis Elimination, Centers for Disease Control and Prevention. TB Notes 1996; 3:25.

16. Raviglione MC, Snider DE Jr, Kochi A. Global epidemiology of tuberculosis. Morbidity and mortality of a worldwide epidemic. JAMA 1995; 273:220-6. Nowak R. WHO calls for action against TB. Science 1995; 267:1763.

17. Dolin PJ, Raviglione MC, Kochi A. Estimates of the future of global tuberculosis morbidity and mortality. Morbidity and Mortality

Weekly Report 1993; 42:961-4. Dolin PJ, Raviglione MC, Kochi A. Global tuberculosis incidence and mortality during 1990-2000. Bull World Health Org 1994; 72:213-20.

Chapter 7: Etude

1. Belloc H. Complete verse: Including sonnets and verse, cautionary verses, the modern traveller, etc; with a preface by W.N. Rougehead. London: Gerald Duckworth, 1970.

2. Long ER. A history of the therapy of tuberculosis and the case of Frédéric Chopin. Lawrence, KS: University of Kansas Press, 1956. Dubos R, Dubos J. The white plague. Tuberculosis, man, and society. Boston: Little, Brown and Company, 1952. Chopin has many biographers, and there are significant disparities in the details of his life as provided by these various authors. In constructing this chapter, I have relied heavily upon the letters of Chopin himself and of George Sand, who lived with him for many years in Mallorca and Paris. In fact, I have quoted freely and extensively from these letters, letting them reveal the narrative. Among biographers, I have chiefly used the account of Long. Long was a preeminent physician scientist and student of tuberculosis. His account of Chopin's illness fits well with what is known about the pathogenesis of the disease. The best known account of Chopin's tuberculosis may be that of René and Jean Dubos. However, when discrepancies between the Dubos and the Long accounts occur, the Long accounts are more consistent with the letters of Chopin and Sand and with the known pathogenesis of tuberculosis.

3. Opienski H. Chopin's Letters. Translated from the original Polish and French. New York: Alfred A. Knopf, 1931. Subsequent quotations from the letters of Chopin in this chapter are from the same source.

4. Sand G. George Sand and Chopin. A glimpse of Bohemia (a letter written to M. Francois Rollinat dated March 8, 1839; translated by Lewis Buddy). Canton, PA: The Kirgate Press, 1902. Subsequent quotations from this letter by Sand in this chapter are from the same source.

5. As noted, Chopin and Sand, both nominally Catholics, did not attend mass.

6. Sand's use of the word wheelbarrow to describe the conveyance

they used is interesting, but it is certain that their exodus was not made using a wheelbarrow. The now archaeic Spanish word *birlocho* describes a two, or occasionally four-wheeled, cart drawn by a horse or mule in which the passengers sit on benches facing each other, and in two other more detailed descriptions of the departure from Valdemosa Sand describes the birlocho as a "sorte de cabriolet à quatre places," a two-wheeled, horse-drawn vehicle seating four people: Sand G. Un Hiver a Majorque—Spiridion. Paris: Michel Levy Freres, 1869:101; and Godeau M. Le Voyage à Majorque de George Sand et Frédéric Chopin. Paris: Nouvelle Editions Debresse, 1959:98-99. Sand G. Correspondance. Tome IV (Mai 1837—Mars 1840). Paris: Garnier Freres, 1968:582-586. The French word for wheelbarrow, *brouette*, is used only in this shorter account, probably for dramatic effect.

7. Dr. Clark also attended Keats (see Chapter 12).

8. It is not clear from my research whether the Dr. Cruveilhier who attended Chopin at his death in Paris is the same as the Dr. Cauvière, whom Georges Sand stated cared for Chopin in Marseilles after their departure from Mallorca.

Chapter 8: Amimalcula

1. Frascatorius H. The theory of infection. In Major RH. Classic descriptions of disease with biographical sketches of the authors, third edition. Springfield, IL: Charles C. Thomas, 1945:7-9.

2. Fomes (singular), fomites (plural) is an old medical term rooted in the Latin word for tinder (see Appendix II). As used by Frascatorius, it probably meant any object transmitting infection by being in contact first with a diseased person and then with a susceptible individual. As used today, it specifically refers to inanimate objects on or in which infectious particles are trapped in adherent dust or on surfaces. The term is not usually used to include airborne infectious particles.

3. Major RH. Op. cit. Meachen GN. A short history of tuberculosis. London: Staples Press Limited, 1936; Gordon BL. Medieval and renaissance medicine. New York: Philosophical Library, 1959:474-80. Myers JA. Captain of all these men of death. Tuberculosis historical highlights. St. Louis: Warren H. Green, Inc., 1977.

4. Defoe D. Journal of the plague year, being observations or memorials of the most remarkable occurrences as well publick as private, which happened in London during the last great vistation in 1665, 1722. Major RH. Op cit:91-3. Major discusses Defoe's comments in the context of the history of infectious disease concepts.

5. Major RH. Op cit:58-62.

6. Doetsch RN. Benjamin Marten and his "New Theory of Consumptions." Microbiol Rev 1978; 42:521-28. Martens' paper and work are discussed by a number of medical historians. I have relied chiefly on Doetsch.

7. Laennec RTH. A treatise on the diseases of the chest, translated by John Forbes. New York: Hafner Publishing Company, 1962. Comroe JH Jr. Retrospectoscope. T.B. or not T. B. Part I. The cause of tuberculosis. Am Rev Respir Dis 1978; 117:137-43. Forbes's translation has been criticized by Comroe for its extensive reorganization of the text. Comroe's criticisms do not detract from the essential lucidity and importance of Laennec's treatise. Gaspard Laurant Bayle, who like Laennec died of tuberculosis, published an earlier description of 900 autopsies of tuberculosis victims. His descriptions and interpretations were criticized by Laennec, but they both came to the important conclusion that tuberculosis in its various forms in different parts of the body represented a single disease.

8. Myers JA. Op cit.

9. Major RH. Op cit:66-68.

10. Myers JA. Op cit:28-30.

11. Meachen CN. Op cit:65.

12. Judge JK. Henry Norman Bethune, M.D. (1890-1939). The T.B.'s progress. J Lab Clin Med 1987; 110:125-6. Dr. Judge wrote this interesting account while a medical student at Case Western Reserve University.

Chapter 9: Robert Koch and the Tubercle Bacillus

1. Brock TD. Robert Koch. A life in medicine and bacteriology. New York: Springer-Verlag, 1988. There is a surprising paucity of biographical material about Koch. Brock has written the only major En-

glish language biography of Koch; it is excellent. Brock brings to the work his own background in microbiology. Moreover, the book is highly readable. I have relied heavily upon Brock's account. Carter KC. Essays of Robert Koch. New York: Greenwood Press, 1987. The introductory section of Carter's collection of several of Koch's major papers in English translation provides much useful biographical information, upon which I have also relied. Sakula A. Robert Koch (1843-1910): Founder of the science of bacteriology and discoverer of the tubercle bacillus. A study of his life and work. Brit J Dis Chest 1979; 73:389-94). Grange JM, Bishop PJ. "Uber tuberkulose." A tribute to Robert Koch's discovery of the tubercle bacillus, 1882. Tubercle 1982; 63:3-17. The papers by Sakula and by Grange and Bishop provide short biographical accounts together with comments on Koch's work.

2. Brock TD. Op cit:24.

3. *Bacillus anthracis.* The word bacillus is often used in this chapter and elsewhere in its general sense to indicate a germ or bacterium. *Bacillus* is also the name of a genus of microorganisms that are rod-shaped, have certain staining characteristics, and form spores. The anthrax bacillus is a member of this genus, and its proper Linnean name is *Bacillus anthracis.*

4. Carter KC. Op cit:xiii-xiv.

5. Sakula A. Op cit. Brock TD, Op cit:116.

6. Most of the bacteria that are common in our environment and with which we are all familiar have generation times of the order of twenty to thirty minutes. That is, each germ divides to produce two new germs each twenty to thirty minutes. As a result, cultures used by doctors to identify these germs are mature and contain a sufficient number of bacteria so that they can be examined to identify the organism within twelve to twenty-four hours. Tubercle bacilli have a generation time of about twenty to twenty-four hours. That means that it takes several weeks for a culture to mature sufficiently so that it can be studied.

7. Carter KC. Op cit:xvi.

8. Koch R. Die aetiologie der tuberculose, a translation by Berna Pinner and Max Pinner with an introduction by Allen K. Krause. Am Rev Tuberc 1932; 25:285-323.

9. *Mycobacterium tuberculosis.* The proper Linnean scientific name

for the tubercle bacillus. This name was not used by Koch, but it is used by all microbiologists today. The tubercle bacillus was originally named *Bacillus tuberculosis*; it is rod-shaped like other members of the genus *Bacillus*, and Koch and other early bacteriologists interpreted its metachromatic staining property as a manifestation of spore formation. Several years later it was recognized not to be a spore-former, and its distinctive wax-like lipids became the basis for its generic name.

10. Koch R. Op cit: 306.

11. Cited by . Carter KC. Op cit:xvi.

12. Ibid.

13. Grange JM, Bishop PJ. Op cit.

14. Trudeau EL. An autobiography. New York: Doubleday, Doran and Company, Inc., 1944:175.

15. *Vibrio cholera*. Linnean name for the cholera bacillus.

16. Brock TD. Op cit:180.

17. Burke DS. Of postulates and peccadilloes: Robert Koch and vaccine (tuberculin) therapy for tuberculosis. Vaccine 1993; 11:795-804.

18. Koch R. A further communication on a remedy for tuberculosis. Deutsche Medicinische Wochenschrift, November 15, 1890. English translation published in Brit Med J, November 22, 1890:1193-5.

19. Koch and his critics. JAMA 1891; 16:59.

20. Burke DS. Op cit.

21. Ibid.

22. Cited by Burke DS, op cit, and Brock TC, op cit:300.

23. Brock TD. Op cit:223-9.

24. There is an apocryphal story, which I have not been able to confirm, that Ehrlich made his personal diagnosis of tuberculosis by staining his own sputum.

Chapter 10: A Distinctly Preventable Disease

1. Winslow C-EA. The life of Hermann M. Biggs, M.D., D.Sc., LL.D. Physician and statesman of the public health. Philadelphia: Lea & Feiberger, 1929:86-8. The three consultants who authored this report were Hermann M. Biggs, T. Mitchell Prudden, and Henry P. Loomis.

2. Corrosive sublimate is bichloride of mercury (mercuric chloride), a commonly used antiseptic. How one would burn a solution of this salt in water is a question that boggles the modern mind.

3. The human variety of tubercle bacillus infects humans, other primates, and guinea pigs. The bovine variety infects cattle, other large mammals, and rabbits. There are related species of mycobacteria that produce tuberculosis in birds, fish, amphibians, rodents, and some other animals, but they do not generally infect people. Dogs and cats are not very susceptible to tuberculosis. Even at the time this circular was written, many of these limitations on the species range of the infectivity of tubercle bacilli were known; the authors' zeal appears to have overcome their science and objectivity.

4. Winslow C-EA. Op cit:87-8.

5. Winslow C-EA. Op cit:139.

6. Teller ME. The tuberculosis movement. A public health campaign in the progressive era. New York: Greenwood Press, 1988:70.

7. Rosencrantz BG. The trouble with bovine tuberculosis. Bull Hist Med 1985; 59:155-75. Many authors discuss the public health campaigns against bovine tuberculosis. Rosencrantz's is noteworthy as both scholarly and readable.

8. Riley RL, O'Grady F. Airborne infection. Transmission and control. New York: The MacMillan Company, 1961. This work presents an excellent discussion of the emergence of the concepts of airborne infections.

9. Riley RL, Mills CC, Nyka W, Weinstock N, Storey PB, Sultan LU, Riley MC, Wells WF. Aerial dissemination of pulmonary tuberculosis. A two-year study of contagion in a tuberculosis ward. Am J Hyg 1959; 70:185-96.

10. Hyge TV. Epidemic of tuberculosis in a state school, with an observation period of about 3 years. Acta Tuberc Scand 1947; 21:1-57.

11. Chapman JS, Dyerly MD. Intrafamilial transmission of tuberculosis. Am Rev Respir Dis 1964; 90:48-60.

12. National Tuberculosis Association. Infectiousness of tuberculosis. Am Rev Respir Dis 1967; 96:836-7.

13. Kline SE, Hedemark LL, Davies SF. Outbreak of tuberculosis among regular patrons of a neighborhood bar. New Engl J Med 1995; 333:222-7.

14. Braden CR, Investigative Team. Infectiousness of a university student with laryngeal and cavitary tuberculosis. Clin Infect Dis 1995; 21:565-70.

15. MacIntyre CR, Plant AJ, Hulls J, Streeton JA, Graham NMH, Rouch GJ. High rate of transmission of tuberculosis in an office: Impact of delayed diagnosis. Clin Infect Dis 1995; 21:1170-4.

16. Driver CR, Valway SE, Morgan WM, Onorato IM, Castro KG. Transmission of *Mycobacterium tuberculosis* associated with air travel. JAMA 1994; 272:1031-1035. Centers for Disease Control. Exposure of passengers and flight crews to *Mycobacterium tuberculosis* on commercial aircraft, 1992-1995. MMWR 1995; 44:137-40.

Chapter 11: Heroes

1. These four vignettes all describe patients whom I cared for personally as a physician.

2. There have been many studies published documenting the high tuberculosis case rates experienced by medical and nursing students during the first half of this century. Among them: Lees HD. Tuberculosis in medical students and nurses. JAMA 1951; 147:1754-7. Barrett-Connor E. The epidemiology of tuberculosis in physicians. JAMA 1979; 241:33-8.

Chapter 12: Two Men of Letters

1. Psalm 23:4. The Holy Bible. Revised Standard Version. New York: Thomas Nelson and Sons, 1953.

2. Stevenson RL. A child's garden of verses. New York: Charles Scribner's Sons, 1905.

3. Hale-White W. Keats as doctor and patient. London: Oxford University Press, 1938. Hewlett D. A life of John Keats. New York: Barnes and Noble, Inc., 1970. Many biographies of Keats have been published, and it is interesting that there are discrepancies among them with regard to factual matters. There is even no agreement on the date of his birth! I have relied heavily, but not exclusively, on these two. Both

works are scholarly. Hale-White's account of Keats's illness is the most consistent of several such works I have reviewed with modern knowledge of the pathogenesis of tuberculosis.

4. Hale-White W. Op cit.

5. Ibid.

6. Wells WA. A doctor's life of John Keats. New York: Vantage Press, 1959:1198-9.

7. It may be recalled that Clark also treated Chopin.

8. Hale-White W. Op cit.

9. Hewlett D. Op cit.

10. Ibid.

11. Moorman LJ. Tuberculosis and genius. Chicago: The University of Chicago Press, 1940. Rice RA. Robert Louis Stevenson. How to know him. Indianapolis, IN: The Bobbs-Merrill Company, 1916. Winchester S. A century after his death, everyone seems to love RLS. Smithsonian 1995; 26(5):50-9. Although there have been many biographies of Robert Louis Stevenson, few have given serious consideration to his illness. I have relied heavily on Moorman. Moorman's account not only details the chronic and relapsing course of Stevenson's disease, but it provides information that makes it possible to relate his illness to tuberculosis as we understand the disease pathogenesis today.

12. Rothman SM. Living in the shadow of death. Tuberculosis and the social experience of illness in American history. New York: Basic Books, 1994. This readable and scholarly work includes accounts of the life of many patients with tuberculosis who sought benefit from a wilderness sojurn in the American West.

13. Chalmers S. The penny piper of Saranac. Boston: Houghton Mifflin Boston, 1916.

14. Trudeau EL. An autobiography. New York: Doubleday, Doran, and Company, Inc., 1944:183.

15. Moorman EL. Op cit:29.

16. Zeidberg LD, Gass RS, Dillon A, Hutcheson RH. The Williamson County tuberculosis study. A twenty-four-year epidemiologic study. Am Rev Respir Dis 1963; 87(suppl):1-88. The most convincing evidence for the effects of age upon the expression of tuberculosis are the data collected in Williamson County, Tennessee in the pretreatment era. The study was shepherded by Wade Hampton Frost; see Chapter 5 for an

account of his seminal contribution to the understanding of the epidemiology of tuberculosis.

Chapter 13: A Brownish Transparent Liquid

1. Koch, R. On Bacteriological Research. Translated by K. Codell Carter and published in Carter KC. Essays of Robert Koch. New York: Greenwood Press, 1987.

2. Koch R. A further communication on a remedy for tuberculosis. Originally published in Deutsche Medicinische Wochenschrift, an English translation was published by the British Medical Journal on November 22, 1890 as a special supplement to the issue of November 15, 1890.

3. Burke DS. Of postulates and peccadilloes: Robert Koch and vaccine (tuberculin) therapy for tuberculosis. Vaccine 1993; 11:795-804.

4. Myers JA. Tuberculosis. A half century of study and conquest. St. Louis: Warren H. Green, Inc., 1970. Edwards PQ, Edwards LB. Story of the tuberculin test from an epidemiologic viewpoint. Am Rev Respir Dis 1960; 81(suppl):1-47. Snider DE Jr. The tuberculin skin test. Am Rev Respir Dis 1982; 125 (suppl):108-18. The story of the development of diagnostic tuberculin testing and its early use by veterinarians has been told in readable fashion by these and other authors.

5. Myers JA, Steele JH. Bovine tuberculosis control in man and animals. St. Louis: Warren H. Green, Inc. 1969:74-5.

6. Turk JL. Von Pirquet, allergy and infectious diseases: a review. J Roy Soc Med 1987; 80:31-3.

7. Bendiner E. Baron von Pirquet: The aristocrat who discovered and defined allergy. Hospital Practice 1981; 16(10):137-58.

8. von Pirquet C. Frequency of tuberculosis in childhood. JAMA 1909; 52:675-8.

9. Pathologists introduced the term miliary tuberculosis to describe tuberculosis that has been widely disseminated throughout the body via the blood stream. The small lesions seen at autopsy were thought to resemble millet seeds. This form of tuberculosis, to which infected infants and young children are particularly susceptible, is invariably fatal in the absence of effective drug therapy.

10. Welch also recruited Wade Hampton Frost to Johns Hopkins University (Chapter 5).

11. Founded by Dr. Lawrence F. Flick (Chapter 21).

12. Daniel TM. Soluble mycobacterial antigens, in Kubica GP, Wayne LG, editors. The mycobacteria: A sourcebook. New York: Marcel Dekker, Inc., 1984:417-65.

13. Edwards LB, Acquaviva FA, Livesay VT, Cross FW, Palmer CE. An atlas of sensitivity to tuberculin, PPD-B, and histoplasmin in the United States. Am Rev Respir Dis 1969; 99 (suppl):1-132. This classical work still provides epidemiologic information of great importance to physicians working in the field of tuberculosis and related infections.

Chapter 14: A Family Affair

1. Long ER. Obituary. Max B. Lurie 1893-1966. Am Rev Respir Dis 1967; 95:694-6. Additional biographical information was obtained from a newspaper obituary clipping dated September 25, 1966, the source of which is not identifiable, and a completed faculty biographical questionnaire dated September 30, 1955, both provided by the University of Pennsylvania Archives.

2. Newspaper obituary. Op. cit.

3. Founded by Dr. Lawrence F. Flick, one of the early proponents of the sanatorium treatment of tuberculosis and advocates for research on tuberculosis. See Chapter 21.

4. Lurie MB. Resistance to tuberculosis. Cambridge, Massachusetts: Harvard University Press, 1964. Lurie's remarkable series of studies was reported in many scientific papers and summarized in this elegant book that is "must reading" for every student of the immunopathogenesis of tuberculosis.

5. Lurie MB. Op. cit:9.

6. Skameme E. Genetic control of susceptibility to mycobacterial infections. Rev Infect Dis 1989; 11(suppl):S394-9.

7. Vidal S, Trembley M, Govoni C, Cauthier S, et al. The Ity/Lsh/Bcg locus: Natural resistance to infection with intracellular parasites is abrogated by disruption of the Nrampl gene. J Exp Med 1995; 182:655-66.

8. Comstock GW. Tuberculosis in twins. A re-analysis of the Prophit survey. Am Rev Respir Dis 1978; 117:621-4.

9. The reduction from 415 to 202 twin pairs in Comstock's analysis was carefully detailed in his paper and appears justified and well reasoned. Among the exclusions were 172 twin pairs in which one of the twins had died in infancy of nontuberculous causes.

10. Stead WW, Senner JW, Reddick WT, Lofgren JP. Racial differences in susceptibility to infection by Mycobacterium tuberculosis. New Engl J Med 1990; 322:422-7.

11. Hoge CW, Fisher L, Donnell HD Jr, Dodson DR, et al. Risk factors for transmission of *Mycobacterium tuberculosis* in a primary school outbreak: Lack of racial difference in susceptibility to infection. Am J Epidemiol 1994; 139:520-30.

12. Katz J, Kunofsky S. Environmental versus constitutional factors in the development of tuberculosis among negroes. Am Rev Respir Dis 1960; 81:17-25.

13. Crowle AJ, Elkins N. Relative permissiveness of macrophages from black and white people for virulent tubercle bacilli. Infect Immun 1990; 58:632-8.

14. Rich AR. The pathogenesis of tuberculosis, second edition. Springfield, IL: Charles C. Thomas, 1944.

15. Bates JH, Stead WW. The history of tuberculosis as a global epidemic. Med Clin North Amer 1993; 77:1205-17. The subject is carefully reviewed by Bates and Stead in this very readable account that includes references to many sources that are not easily found elsewhere.

16. Cummins LS. Tuberculosis in primitive tribes and its bearing on the tuberculosis of civilized communities. Internat J Public Health 1920; 1:137-71.

17. Borrel A. Pneumonie et tuberculose chez les troupes noire. Ann Inst Pasteur 1920; 34:105-48.

18. Stead WW, Eisenach KD, Cave MD, Beggs ML, et al. When did *Mycobacterium tuberculosis* infection first occur in the new world? An important question with public health implications. Am J Respir Crit Care Med 1995; 151:1267-8. In communications with the authors of that article, I and Jacques Grosset have both challenged the conclusions of this paper. I felt that the hypothesis that *M. tuberculosis* evolved from *M. bovis* or any other currently extant form was inconsistent with gen-

eral precepts of biology. Grosset felt on the basis of his virulence studies that *M. bovis* is probably a more recently evolved organism than *M. tuberculosis*. He further felt that the diversity of *M. tuberculosis* strains seen in Africa argues for the presence of tubercle bacilli on this continent at a much earlier date than that accepted by these authors. Youmans GP. Tuberculosis. Philadelphia: W.B. Saunders Company, 1979:362-3. Youmans, a distinguished microbiologist who devoted his life to the study of tuberculosis, argues forcefully that even in populations with the highest tuberculosis death rates that can logically be accepted, the selection pressure would not be great enough to lead to the evolution of a resistant population.

19. Shakespeare W. Hamlet, Prince of Denmark: act 5, scene 2, lines 10-11. William Shakespeare. The complete works. London: Collins, 1951. There's a divinity that shapes our ends, rough-hew them how we will.

Chapter 15: Bacille Calmette-Guérin

1. Clendening L. Source book of medical history. New York: Paul B. Hoebler, Inc., 1942:291-305.

2. Ibid.

3. Clendening, op. cit:388-92. Vallery-Radot R. The life of Pasteur. New York: Doubleday, Page and Company, 1919:414-7. Geison GL. The private science of Louis Pasteur. Princeton, NJ: Princeton University Press, 1995. Geison discusses the debate which occurred at the time and has persisted over Pasteur's absence of statistical data, lack of a planned trial, and possible disregard of ethical considerations as he treated Meister and others.

4. Koch R. Weitere Mitteilunger uber ein Heilmittel gegen Tuberculose. Dtsch Med Wschr 1891; 17:101-2. Translated and quoted in Bothamley GH, Grange JM. The Koch phenomenon and delayed hypersensitivity: 1891-1991. Tubercle 1991; 72:7-11.

5. Sakula A. BCG: Who were Calmette and Guérin? Thorax 1983; 38:806-12. Bendiner E. Albert Calmette: A vaccine and its vindication. Hospital Practice (Office Ed) Oct 1992; 27(10A):113-6,119-22,125,129-32. Both sources provide highly readable and detailed accounts of Calmette's life and achievements.

6. Sakula A. Op. cit.

7. Sakula A, op. cit. and Bendiner E, op. cit. Bloom BR, Fine PEM. Chapter 31. The BCG experience: Implications for future vaccines against tuberculosis. In Bloom BR, editor. Tuberculosis: Pathogenesis, protection, and control. Washington: American Society for Microbiology, 1994:531-57. The story of Calmette's and Guérin's work is recounted in these two works.

8. Sakula A, op. cit. Bloom BR and Fine PEM, op. cit. Accounts of this first use of BCG vary somewhat in minor details. I have relied chiefly on these two sources. Calmette and Guérin believed that the natural route of infection in humans for bovine strains of tubercle bacilli, such as the one from which their vaccine was developed, was oral. For this reason, they administered their vaccine orally. Later, inoculation into the skin became the preferred and much more convenient route. There are, however, some arcane reasons based on modern immunology to believe that oral immunization against tuberculosis might be better than intracutaneous vaccination. None of the many controlled scientific evaluations of BCG have used the oral route, however.

9. Sakula A. Op cit.

10. Feldberg GD. Disease and class. Tuberculosis and the shaping of modern North American society. New Brunswick, NJ: Rutgers University Press, 1995:126.

11. Calmette A. Epilogue de la catastrophe de Lubeck. La Presse Médicale 1931; 39:17-8.

12. For the third time, we note that the Phipps Institute was founded by Lawrence F. Flick, whom we will meet in Chapter 21. A physician, Flick, like Edward Livingston Trudeau, who founded the famous sanatorium in Saranac Lake, was remarkable for recognizing the importance that science might contribute to the conquest of tuberculosis.

13. Aronson JD, Aronson CF, Taylor HC. A twenty-year appraisal of BCG vaccination in the control of tuberculosis. Arch Int Med 1958; 101:881-93.

14. Comstock GW. The international tuberculosis campaign: A pioneering venture in mass vaccination and research. Clin Infect Dis 1994; 19:528-40. The story of Holm's remarkable leadership in mounting the postwar tuberculosis control program in Europe is told in readable fashion by Dr. Comstock, the dean of American tuberculosis epidemiolo-

gists, who draws on his personal knowledge of the events and people involved. See also Chapter 5. I recall vividly a conversation that I had with Holm after a tuberculosis control planning meeting in Ghana in 1971; Holm emphasized the need to move forcefully in initiating programs without waiting for the approvals of all layers of officialdom.

15. Comstock GW, Webster RG. Tuberculosis studies in Muscogee County, Georgia. VII. A twenty-year evaluation of BCG vaccination in a school population. Am Rev Respir Dis 1969; 100:839-45.

16. Feldberg GD. Op. cit.

17. Ibid:175.

18. Tuberculosis Vaccines Clinical Trials Committee. B.C.G. and vole bacillus vaccines in the prevention of tuberculosis in adolescence and early adult life. Brit Med J 1963; 1:973-978.

19. Dubos R. The J. Burns Amberson lecture. Acquired immunity to tuberculosis. Am Rev Respir Dis 1964; 90:505-15.

20. It is reasonable to suppose that the disparate results obtained in trials of BCG efficacy might be due to strain differences, and some experts believe this to be the case. On the other hand, there is also a substantial body of scientific opinion that believes that this is not an adequate explanation for the differences found. The only trial specifically designed to address this question was the South India trial, but since no protection was observed, no information on strain differences can be extracted from the results.

21. WHO Expert Committee on Tuberculosis. Ninth Report. Technical Report Series No. 552. Geneva: World Health Organization, 1974:26.

22. Fine PEM. The BCG story: Lessons from the past and implications for the future. Rev Infect Dis 1989; 11(suppl):S353-9.

23. Tuberculosis Prevention Trial. Trial of BCG vaccines in south India for tuberculosis prevention: First report. Bull World Health Org 1979; 57:819-27. Tuberculosis Prevention Trial, Madras. Trial of BCG vaccines in south India for tuberculosis prevention. Indian J Med Res 1979; 70:349-63.

24. Tripathy SP. Fifteen-year follow-up of the Indian BCG prevention trial. Bull Internat Union against Tuberc 1987; 62(3):69-72. Tripathy SP. Ann Natl Med Sci (India) 1983; 19:1-21.

25. Colditz GA, Brewer TF, Berkey CS, Wilson ME, et al. Efficacy of

BCG vaccine in the prevention of tuberculosis. Meta-analysis of the published literature. JAMA 1994; 271:698-702. Comstock GW. Field trials of tuberculosis vaccines: How could we have done them better? Controlled Clin Trials 1994; 15:247-76. Both sources provide excellent summaries of this field; that of Comstock is perhaps more complete.
26. Comstock GW. Op. cit.

Chapter 16: Four Cornerposts of Science

1. Chase MW. Immunity and experimental dermatology. Ann Rev Immunol 1995; 3:1-29. Chase MW. Early days in cellular immunology. Allergy Proc 1988; 9:683-7. My account is based on these two historical review articles written by Dr. Chase and on several conversations and personal correspondence with Dr. Chase, whom it has been my great privilege and pleasure to know.

2. Chase MW. The cellular transfer of cutaneous hypersensitivity to tuberculin. Proc Soc Exper Biol Med 1945; 59:134-5.

3. Bates B. Bargaining for life. A social history of tuberculosis, 1876-1938. Philadelphia: University of Pennsylvania Press, 1992:119-22.

4. Pearmain G, Lycette RR, Fitzgerald PH. Tuberculin-induced mitosis in peripheral blood leucocytes. Lancet 1963; 1:637-8.

5. Schrek R. Cell transformations and mitoses produced in vitro by tuberculin purified protein derivative in human blood cells. Am Rev Respir Dis 1963; 87:734-8.

6. Hinz CF Jr, Daniel TM, Baum GL. Quantitative aspects of the stimulation of lymphocytes by tuberculin purified protein derivative. Int Arch Allerg and Immunol 1970; 38:119-29.

7. David JR. Delayed hypersensitivity in vitro: Its mediation by cell-free substances formed by lymphoid cell-antigen interaction. Proc Nat Acad Sc 1966; 56:72-7.

8. Bloom BR, Bennet B. Mechanism of a reaction in vitro associated with delayed-type hypersensitivity. Science 1966; 153:80-2.

9. Good RA. The dual immunity systems and resistance to infection. Medicine 1973; 52:405-10. Culliton BJ. Immunology: Two immune systems capture attention. Science 1973; 180:45-8,89. The story of the discovery of separate T- and B-lymphocyte mediated immune

responses is related in readable fashion in these two articles.

10. The account of Warren's work is based not only on his many published papers but also on my personal knowledge. Dr. Warren and I were friends and classmates at Harvard Medical School as well as faculty colleagues in the Department of Medicine at Case Western Reserve University.

11. Hang LM, Warren KS, Boros DL. *Schistosoma mansoni*: Antigenic secretions and the etiology of egg granulomas in mice. Exper Parasit 1974; 35:288-98. Among Warren's many published papers, the review provided in this paper is particularly helpful.

12. Boros DL, Warren KS. The bentonite granuloma. Characterization of a model system for infectious and foreign body granulomatous inflammation using soluble mycobacterial, histoplasma and schistosoma antigens. Immunol 1973; 24:511-29. The soluble mycobacterial antigens used in this study were provided by my laboratory.

Chapter 17: The Cursed Duet

1. Corbitt G, Bailey AS, Williams G. HIV infection in Manchester, 1959. Lancet 1990; 2:51.

2. Centers for Disease Control. *Pneumocystis carinii* pneumonia—Los Angeles. Morbidity Mortality Weekly Report 1981; 30:250-2. Centers for Disease Control. Kaposi's sarcoma and *Pneumocystis carinii* pneumonia among homosexual men—New York City and California. Morbidity Mortality Weekly Report 1981; 30:305-8.

3. Serwadda D, Mugerwa RD, Sewankambo NK, Lwegaba A, et al. Slim disease: a new disease in Uganda and its association with HTLV-III infection. Lancet 1985; 2:849-852.

4. Sunderam G, McDonald RJ, Maniatis T, Oleske J, Kapila R, Reichman LB. Tuberculosis as a manifestation of the acquired immunodeficiency syndrome (AIDS). JAMA 1986; 256:362-6.

5. Pitchenik AE, Rubinson HA. The radiographic appearance of tuberculosis in patients with the acquired immune deficiency syndrome AIDS and pre-AIDS. Am Rev Respir Dis 1985; 131:393-6.

6. Goodgame RW. AIDS in Uganda—clinical and social features. New Engl J Med 1990; 323:383-9.

7. Sunderam, et al. Op. Cit.

8. Chrétien J. Tuberculosis and HIV. The cursed duet. Bull Internat Union against Tuberc 1990; 65:25-8.

9. Dolin PJ, Raviglione MC, Kochi A. Global tuberculosis incidence and mortality during 1990-2000. Bull World Health Org 1994; 72:213-220.

Chapter 18: Victories

1. Milne, AA. Now we are six. New York: E.P. Dutton & Co., Inc., 1927.

2. Marble A, with Leatherman D. Courting danger. New York: St. Martin's Press, 1991. All of the biographical material and the associated quotations in this chapter are taken from this posthumously published autobiography.

3. Pottenger FM. Tuberculosis. A discussion of phthisiogenesis, immunology, pathologic physiology, diagnosis, and treatment. St. Louis: C.V. Mosby Company, 1948.

4. Pottenger FM, op. cit:394-5.

5. Marble A., op. cit.

6. Pottenger FM, op. cit:321-2.

7. Baker J, Bouillon J. Josephine. New York: Harper & Row Publishers, Inc., 1977.

8. Ibid.

9. Grzybowski S, Enarson DA. The fate of cases of pulmonary tuberculosis under various treatment programmes. Bull Internat Union Against Tuberc 1978; 53:7-75.

Chapter 19: Wolf's Liver and Sea Voyages

1. Sledzik PS, Bellantoni N. Brief communication: Bioarcheological and biocultural evidence for the New England vampire folk belief. Am J Phys Anthropology 1994; 94:269-74.

2. Ibid.

3. Long ER. A history of the therapy of tuberculosis and the case of

Frédéric Chopin. Lawrence, KS: University of Kansas Press, 1956:43-4.

4. Long ER. Op. cit:39.

5. Clendening L. Source book of medical history. New York: Paul B. Hoeber, 1942:84.

6. Bates B. Bargaining for life. A social history of tuberculosis, 1876-1938. Philadelphia: University of Pennsylvania Press, 1992:215.

7. Pottenger FM. Tuberculosis. A discussion of phthisiogenesis, immunology, pathologic physiology, diagnosis, and treatment. St. Louis: C.V. Mosby Company, 1948:428.

8. Badger TL. Looking backward. Medical Dimensions 1976 (June):8-11.

9. Clendinning L. Op. cit:434.

10. Meckel RA. Open-air schools and the tuberculous child in early 20th-century America. Arch Pediatr Adolesc Med 1996; 150:91-5.

11. Badger TL. Op. cit.

12. Bercher J. Los Curanderos. La Présse Medicale, April 1939. Cited by Dubos R, Dubos J. The white plague. Tuberculosis, man, and society. New Brunswick, NJ: Rutgers University Press, 1987:256. Gallagher R. Diseases that plague modern man. A history of ten communicable diseases. Dobbs Ferry, NY: Oceana Publications, Inc., 1969:168. The same episode is described by Gallagher without a source citation as by Dubos and Dubos. The Dubos's account was originally published in 1952, and it is likely that Gallagher took his account from their book.

13. Long ER. Op. cit:45.

14. Rothman SM. Living in the shadow of death. Tuberculosis and the social experience of illness in American history. New York: HarperCollins Publishers, 1994.

Chapter 20: False Hope

1. Koch R. Ueber bakteriologische Forschung. Verhandlungen des X Internationalen Medizinischen Kongresses. Berlin: August Hirschwald, 1890. Translated and published in Carter CC. Essays of Robert Koch. Westport, CT: Greenwood Press, Inc., 1987:179-86. Burke DS. Of postulates and peccadilloes: Robert Koch and vaccine (tuberculin)

therapy for tuberculosis. Vaccine 1993; 11:795-804. Burke not only gives an account of this presentation but also of the subsequent events.

2. Koch R. A further communication on a remedy for tuberculosis. British Med J 1890; 2:1193-5.

3. Ibid. See also, Lancet 1890; 2:1085-96.

4. Ibid.

5. Burke DS. Op. cit.

6. Anonymous. British Med J 1890; 2:1195-7.

7. Dubos R, Dubos J. The white plague. Tuberculosis, man, and society. New Brunswick, NJ: Rutgers University Press, 1987:105-107.

8. Burke DS. Op, cit.

9. Anonymous. Lancet 1890; 2:1107-8.

10. Anonymous. Dr. Koch's investigations upon the treatment of tuberculosis. Lancet 1890; 2:932-3.

11. Anonymous. The lay press and medical research. Lancet 1890; 2:1354.

12. Richmond WS. Professor Koch's remedy for tuberculosis. Lancet 1890; 2:1354-5.

13. Anonymous. Professor Koch's treatment of tuberculosis. Lancet 1890; 2:1347-8.

14. Burke DS. Op. cit.

15. Pottenger FM. Tuberculosis. A discussion of phthisiogenesis, immunology, pathologic physiology, diagnosis, and treatment. St. Louis: The C.V. Mosby Company, 1948:437-56.

Chapter 21: Places Apart

1. Mann's experience in Davos is told by him in an appendix to the Vintage International edition of Mann T. The magic mountain, New York: Random House, Inc., 1980.

2. Knopf SA. The centenary of Brehmer's birth. Am Rev Tuberc 1926; 14:207-10. Meachen GN. A short history of tuberculosis. London: Staples Press Limited, 1936:18-9. The priority usually assigned to Brehmer's German sanatorium can be challenged by several institutions in England. The Royal Sea Bathing Infirmary for Scrofula was opened at Margate in 1791; it was later converted to a tuberculosis hospital.

The Royal Hospital for Diseases of the Chest was opened in London in 1814, the Brompton Hospital for Consumption and Diseases of the Chest in 1841, and the City of London Hospital for Diseases of the Chest in 1851, all earlier than Brehmer's sanatorium. However, none of the British facilities provided long term care for tuberculosis patients. The Channing Home in Boston did provide chrronic care for tuberculosis patients beginning two years before Brehmer's sanatorium (see text).

3. Kass AM. Harriet Ryan Albee. Charity begins at the Channing Home. Harvard Medical Alumni Bulletin 1989; 62:48-53. The author of this article was the wife of the late Edward H. Kass, Professor of Medicine at Harvard Medical School, a distinguished academic infectious disease physician-scientist. He served as Director of the Channing Laboratory.

4. Trudeau EL. An autobiography. New York: Doubleday, Doran and Company, Inc., 1944:71.

5. I have relied heavily for biographical material upon Trudeau EL. An autobiography. Op. cit. This very personal account is obviously not an objective assessment of Trudeau's life and work. At the same time, it is an important source for all interested in the history of tuberculosis. The quotations in this chapter, unless otherwise noted, are from this source. Meade GM. Edward Livingston Trudeau, M.D. Tubercle 1972; 53:229-50. Meade presents a concise account of Trudeau's life and work. Tyler HA. The story of Paul Smith. Born smart. Utica, NY: North Country Books, Inc., 1988. This book provides anecdotal accounts of Trudeau's early years at Paul Smith's. Ellison DL. Healing tuberculosis in the woods. Medicine and science at the end of the nineteenth century. Westport, CT: Greenwood Press, 1994. This biography emphasizes Trudeau's contributions to medical science.

6. Trudeau EL. An experimental study of preventive inoculation in tuberculosis. Medical Record (New York) 1890; 38:565-8.

7. Bates B. Bargaining for life. A social history of tuberculosis, 1876-1938. Philadelphia: University of Pennsylvania Press, 1992. Flick's life and career are authoritatively documented by Bates. The accounts of Flick and his work in this chapter rely principally on this source.

8. Bates B. Op. cit:78.

9. Ibid:140. Additional information concerning G. Justice Ewing came from conversations with his descendents.

10. Davis AL. History of the Sanatorium Movement. In Rom WN,

Garay SN, editors. Tuberculosis. New York: Little, Brown and Company, 1996.

11. Fudenberg HH. The dollar benefits of biomedical research: A cost analysis. J Lab Clin Med 1988; 111:6-12.

12. Mann T. The magic mountain. New York: Random House, Inc., 1980.

13. Ibid:182.

14. Rothman SM. Living in the shadow of death. Tuberculosis and the social experience of illness in American history. New York: HarperCollins Publishers, 1994. The important role of tuberculosis in the settling of the American West is treated admirably by Rothman.

15. Alling DW, Bosworth ER. The after history of pulmonary tuberculosis. VI. The first fifteen years following diagnosis. Am Rev Respir Dis 1960; 81:839-49.

16. Diagnostic standards and classification of tuberculosis. New York: National Tuberculosis and Respiratory Disease Association, 1969. Standardized definitions were developed for the classification of tuberculosis by committees of the National Tuberculosis and Respiratory Disease Association (now the American Lung Association) and the American Thoracic Society. The definitions for extent of disease were last published in the 1969 source cited. Tuberculosis was never considered cured, as the potential for relapse always remained, and such terms as inactive and arrested were used and given precise definitions. Subsequent publications by this organization classified tuberculosis only by its infectiousness; the committees that prepared these publications no longer considered extent and activity of disease to be important.

Chapter 22: Collapse and Mutilation

1. Meade GM. Edward Livingston Trudeau, M.D. Tubercle 1972; 53:229-50.

2. Davis AL. History of the sanatorium movement. In Rom WN, Garay SM, editors. Tuberculosis. New York: Little, Brown and Company, 1996:35-54.

3. Brown L. The story of clinical pulmonary tuberculosis. Baltimore, MD: Williams and Wilkins Company, 1941:235-6. Hochberg

LA. Thoracic surgery before the 20th century. New York: Vantage Press, 1960:378-402. Nissen R, Wilson RHL. Pages in the history of chest surgery. Springfield, IL: Charles C. Thomas Publisher, 1960:51-77. Meade RH. A history of thoracic surgery. Springfield, IL: Charles C. Thomas Publisher, 1961:110-41. Gaensler EA. The surgery for pulmonary tuberculosis. In Green GM, Daniel TM, Ball WC Jr, editors. Koch centennial memorial. Am Rev Respir Dis 1982; 125 (suppl):73-84. Naef AP. The story of thoracic surgery. Milestones and pioneers. Toronto: Hogrefe and Huber Publishers, 1990:13-9. Naef AP. The 1900 tuberculosis epidemic—starting point of modern thoracic surgery. Ann Thorac Surg 1993; 55:1375-8. The history of surgical collapse therapies for tuberculosis is told in a number of additional sources. While these various sources are in general agreement on the facts, they provide a variety of interesting perspectives from individuals many of whom were writing of therapies introduced during their years of medical practice.

4. Brown L. Op. cit.

5. Ibid.

6. Hochberg LA. Op. cit:392.

7. Gaensler EA. Op. cit:78-9.

Meade RH. Op. cit:122-4.

8. Reibman J. Phthisis and the arts. In Rom WN, Garay SM, editors. Tuberculosis. New York: Little, Brown and Company, 1996:21-34.

9. Ibid.

10. Meade RH. Op. Cit:125.

11. Meade RH. Op. Cit:126-127.

Chapter 23: Magic Bullet

1. Ryan F. The forgotten plague. How the battle against tuberculosis was won—and lost. Boston, MA: Little, Brown and Company, 1992. This book tells the story of the development of drug treatment for tuberculosis is told in very readable, often gripping fashion.

2. Waksman SA. My life with the microbes. New York: Simon and Schuster, 1954. Waksman's autobiography, which is delightfully writ-

ten and provides rich insights into his person, is the source for most of the biographical material in this chapter. In some of the sections relating to the role of Albert Schatz in the discovery of streptomycin and Shatz litigation against Waksman, the author may be less than candid.

3. Ibid:65.

4. Byron Waksman became a distinguished experimental pathologist.

5. Comroe, JH Jr. Retrospectroscope. Insights into medical discovery. Menlo Park, CA: Von Gehr Press, 1977:71.

6. Schatz A, Bugie E, Waksman SA. Streptomycin, a substance exhibiting antibiotic activity against Gram-positive and Gram-negative bacteria. Proc Exptl Biol Med 1944; 55:66-9. Waksman SA. The conquest of tuberculosis. Berkley, CA: University of California Press, 1964:103-23. Readers should note that Schatz was the first author on the initial description of streptomycin as well as on subsequent related papers.

7. Waksman SA, 1954, op. cit:208-15. An account of that historic presentation and much of Waksman's text.

8. Waksman SA, 1964, op. cit:123-7.

9. Pfuetze, KH, Pyle MM, Hinshaw HC, Feldman WH. The first clinical trial of streptomycin in human tuberculosis. Am Rev Tuberc 1955; 71:752-4. I have relied on this account of this event published ten years later by the physicians involved. Ryan F. Op. cit:236-41. Ryan also describes the first human use of streptomycin. He interviewed Hinshaw nearly fifty years after the event, and he also referred to the published account. Because of the elapsed time, I have chosen to rely on Hinshaw's published accounts rather than his statements to Ryan when discrepancies occur. Hinshaw described to Ryan an additional patient, an elderly man who died of other causes while improving in response to streptomycin. Ryan describes this man as the first person to be given streptomycin.

10. Hinshaw HV, Feldman WH. Streptomycin in the treatment of clinical tuberculosis: A preliminary report. Proceedings of the Staff Meetings of the Mayo Clinic 1945; 20:313-8.

11. Hinshaw HC, Feldman WH, Pfuetze KH. Treatment of tuberculosis with streptomycin. A summary of observations on one hundred cases. JAMA 1946; 132:778-82.

12. Medical Research Council. Streptomycin treatment of pulmonary tuberculosis. B Med J 1948; 2:769-82.

13. Waksman SA, 1954, op. cit:310.

14. Waksman SA, 1954, op. cit:279-85. In this account, Waksman does not identify Schatz by name, although the circumstances cited make it clear that Schatz was the litigant. Ryan F, op. cit. Ryan gives a detailed account of these events, based on interviews with Schatz, that differs in many details from Waksman's account, on which I have relied. The interviews with Schatz were conducted many years after the event and after hardening of Schatz's bitterness. Ryan, of course, did not have the opportunity to obtain similar interviews with the deceased Waksman. With respect to Waksman's share of royalties, it should be noted that current policy of the National Institutes of Health is that at least ten percent of royalties from inventions conceived under its grants should be assigned to the inventor, and many American universities accord an even higher percentage to their faculty inventors. These payments are considered to provide incentives to faculty scientists.

Chapter 24: Microbe Killers

1. Crick B. George Orwell. A life. Boston: Little, Brown and Company. 1980.
Wykes D. A preface to George Orwell. London: Longman, 1987.

2. Crick B. Op. cit:375. Cutaneous reactions of the type experienced by Orwell are recognized toxic manifestations of both PAS and thioacetazone, either of which might have been given to Orwell along with streptomycin. Such reactions are not generally recognized as among streptomycin's toxicity, although it is never possible to be sure that these rare toxic reactions are not the result of almost any drug.

3. Ryan F. The forgotten plague. How the battle against tuberculosis was won—and lost. Boston: Little, Brown and Company, 1992. Ryan recounts the story of the German drug industry in the development of chemotherapeutic agents in fascinating detail.

4. Selikoff IJ, Robitzek EH, Ornstein GG. Treatment of pulmonary tuberculosis with hydrazide derivatives of isonicotinic acid. JAMA 1952; 150:973-80.

5. Ibid.

6. Dawson JJY, Devadatta S, Fox W, Radhakrishna S, et al. A 5-year study of patients with pulmonary tuberculosis in a concurrent comparison of home and sanatorium treatment for one year with isoniazid plus PAS. Bull Wld Hlth Org 1966; 34:533-51.

7. Kamat SR, Dawson JJY, Devadatta S, Fox W, et al. A controlled study of the influence of segregation of tuberculous patients for one year on the attack rate of tuberculosis in a 5-year period in close family contacts in South India. Bull Wld Hlth Org 1966; 34:517-32.

8. Davis AL. History of the sanatorium movement. In Rom WN, Garay SM, editors. Tuberculosis. New York: Little, Brown and Company, NY, 1996:35-54.

9. Fudenberg HH. The dollar benefits of biomedical research: A cost analysis. J Lab Clin Med 1988; 111:6-12.

10. Verbist L, Gyselen A. Antituberculous activity of rifampin *in vitro* and *in vivo* and the concentrations attained in human blood. Am Rev Respir Dis 1968; 98:923-32. Gyselen A, Verbist L, Cosemans J, Lacquet LM, Vandenbergh E. Rifampin and ethambutol in the retreatment of advanced pulmonary tuberculosis. Am Rev Resp Dis 1968; 98:933-43. Daniel TM. Rifampin—A major new chemotherapeutic agent for the treatment of tuberculosis. New Engl J Med 1969; 280:615-6. International readers should note that the drug known as rifampin in North America is generally called rifampicin in other parts of the world.

11. Fox W. Whither short-course chemotherapy. Brit J Dis Chest 1981; 75:331-57.

12. Edwards A. Vivien Leigh. A biography. Simon and Schuster, New York. 1977.

Chapter 25: One One-Hundredth of an Ounce of Prevention

1. Lincoln EM. The effect of antimicrobial therapy on the prognosis of primary tuberculosis in children. Am Rev Tuberc 1954; 69:682-9.

2. Ibid:687.

3. Ferebee SH. Controlled chemoprophylaxis trials in tuberculosis. A general review. Adv Tuberc Res 1970; 17:28-106.

4. Comstock GW. Isoniazid prophylaxis in an undeveloped area.

Am Rev Resp Dis 1962; 86:810-22.

5. Garibaldi RA, Drusin RE, Ferebee SH, Gregg MB. Isoniazid-associated hepatitis. Report of an outbreak. Am Rev Resp Dis 1972; 106:357-65.

6. Comstock GW, Edwards PQ. The competing risks of tuberculosis and hepatitis among adult tuberculin reactors. Am Rev Respir Dis 1975; 111:573-7.

7. Division of Tuberculosis Elimination, Centers for Disease Control and Prevention, United States Public Health Service. TB Notes, 1993 (Fall).

Chapter 26: Hope in Haiti

1. Matthew 4: 14-16. The Holy Bible. Revised Standard Version. New York: Thomas Nelson and Sons, 1953.

2. Details of the early history of International Child Care are based on information provided to me by William K. Cunningham, long time trustee and treasurer of International Child Care.

3. Details of the Haitian tuberculosis problem and Child Care's response to it come from my personal records of many trips to Haiti as a volunteer consultant helping to plan and implement Child Care's programs.

4. Chaisson RE, Clermont HC, Holt EA, Cantave M, et al. Six-month supervised intermittent tuberculosis therapy in Haitian patients with and without HIV infection. Am J Respir Crit Care Med 196; 154:1034-8.

5. Chaisson RE. Directly observed therapy and its alternatives in cost effective program planning. Presentation made at the International Union against Tuberculosis and Lung Disease, North American Region, Second Mid Year Conference, March 1, 1997.

Index